18"

99BB

SOCIAL WORK
AND
MENTAL HEALTH

SOCIAL WORK AND MENTAL HEALTH

Edited by **James W. Callicutt**
Pedro J. Lecca

THE FREE PRESS
A Division of Macmillan Publishing Co., Inc.
NEW YORK

Collier Macmillan Publishers
LONDON

THE FREE PRESS
A Division of Macmillan Publishing Co., Inc.
866 Third Avenue, New York, N. Y. 10022

Collier Macmillan Canada, Inc.

Printed in the United States of America

printing number

1 2 3 4 5 6 7 8 9 10

Library of Congress Cataloging in Publication Data

Main entry under title:

Social work and mental health.

   Includes bibliographies and index.
   1. Psychiatric social work—United States—Addresses,
essays, lectures. I. Callicutt, James W. II. Lecca,
Pedro J.
HV689.S64   1983   362.2′04256   82-71734
ISBN 0-02-905830-9
ISBN 0-02-905850-3 (pbk.)

My role in writing and editing this book was encouraged by my wife, Ann. My contribution is dedicated with love to her and our children, Frances, Cyndie, Jack, and Daniel.

J.W.C.

The unfaltering devotion of my family has made the effort involved in editing and authoring this book possible.

Their love and continuing support give due cause for dedication of my contributions in this book to them: Gina, Peter, Vincent, and Anthony.

P.J.L.

Contents

Foreword

THE HISTORICAL ROOTS of social work practice in the broad field of mental health can be traced to the nineteenth century in America—a history shared with medicine and nursing. More recently, psychiatry and psychology have joined these traditional human service disciplines. Since World War II, psychiatry, clinical psychology, psychiatric nursing, and psychiatric social work have been recognized as the core mental health professions, each with its own expertise, role, and status, on the one hand, and a common concern for the promotion of mental health including the treatment and care of emotionally disturbed individuals, on the other. More than any other specialist, the social worker deals with the family and social environment of the person seeking help, taking a comprehensive casework approach to past history, current milieu, and future prospects of the individual. In a broad range of settings, the social worker is called upon to intervene in crises, to conduct family counseling, and to engage in individual or group psychotherapy.

Over the past twenty years, the United States has witnessed remarkable changes in the amount and variety of services for people with mental and emotional problems. A generation ago, most mental health care was provided by state or local psychiatric hospitals. Today, less than 10 percent of over six million episodes of care are accounted for by state and county mental hospitals. Outpatient psychiatric services provide half of today's therapy, while almost another third takes place in community mental health centers. Social workers are at the forefront of the community mental health movement, which has pioneered in preventive services and social interventions aimed at promoting mental health; these settings emphasize short-term clinical services directed at emergencies or circumscribed problems.

Throughout this book special attention is given to the knowledge and skills needed by social workers if they are to continue their leadership role within the field of mental health. No longer can a social worker be narrowly trained as a psychiatric caseworker engaged primarily in psychotherapy or social casework with an individual patient and the patient's family. The old controversies between specialty training in psychiatric social work and general training in social work and welfare administration have faded as new challenges have emerged. Social workers today are active in administration, planning, research, training, and community organization. All too frequently, however, academic programs fail to prepare the social worker in mental health planning, organizational and community dynamics, fiscal accounting and reporting, staff supervision, research design and implementation, and community public relations, all vital to fulfilling important social work functions.

While no one can hope to become an expert in all the areas now embraced by the social work profession, both student and practitioner can profit greatly from a careful study of the many topics brought together in this volume. Even as this book goes to press, the human services are undergoing a profound shift from federal to state and local financing. While no one can foresee how far the pendulum will swing away from categorical, large-scale federal support of human services to local and regional support and regulation, the general trend is clear. More than ever before, mental health professionals, including social workers, will have to deal with the spectrum of community factors. This book not only provides a good introduction to emerging national issues but also covers in a thorough and original manner a wide variety of topics central to advanced studies and professional practice in social work and the delivery of mental health services.

Wayne H. Holtzman

Preface

DURING THE PAST several decades mental health services have developed into a major component of one of the nation's largest industries, health care. Public interest and controversy regarding mental health programs is related to both fiscal concerns and emotional feelings about mental disorders and handicaps.

While social work has long been an important profession in the mental health arena, this growth precipitated the rapid recruitment and training of new personnel for the mental health field—not only social workers and others engaged in direct patient care, but also administrators, planners, educators, and researchers. Educational institutions devised new or augmented existing curricula to train additional personnel to fill the jobs created by the burgeoning community mental health movement.

The need for the development and dissemination of knowledge in this area has been recognized. Vast quantities of data on mental health have been produced. However, this available information is far beyond the capacity of anyone to assimilate. Moreover, these instructive bits and pieces of information do not necessarily add up to a whole picture. We were impressed by the need for a convenient, comprehensive view of social work and the mental health field as a whole. Furthermore, the inclusion of an historical perspective reflecting the long tradition of social work appeared appropriate. Consequently, we turned to colleagues who are seasoned practitioners and academicians to join us in writing this volume. Our aim was to blend the conceptual/theoretical and the practical in producing a book that would be useful to students and practitioners in social work and other discplines involved in the field of mental health.

The two editors assume equal responsibility for the product. While our individual views were not always identical, we think that the differences were an asset.

We thank our colleagues who offered helpful suggestions, and the contributing authors for their cooperation and patience. The use of gender pronouns in the book is not uniform as a consequence of the style or preference of the contributing authors.

As customary, the editors take responsibility for all errors—but, we hope, too, for making some important points.

JAMES W. CALLICUTT
PEDRO J. LECCA

About the Editors and Contributors

JAMES W. CALLICUTT received his Ph.D from the Florence Heller Graduate School for Advanced Studies in Social Welfare, Brandeis University. He is Professor and Associate Dean, Graduate School of Social Work, the University of Texas at Arlington, Arlington, Texas. His primary professional interests are the substantive areas of mental health, alcohol abuse, and alcoholism. He is active on community, state, and national boards and committees, and is a member of several professional associations. His publications are in the areas of mental health, retardation, and part-time social work education. Dr. Callicutt has served as a program development consultant for and staff member of a variety of mental health agencies including neuropsychiatric hospitals and community mental health centers.

PEDRO J. LECCA received his Ph.D. from the University of Mississippi. He is Professor, Graduate School of Social Work, the University of Texas at Arlington, Arlington, Texas. His studies include post-doctoral work at Baruch College/Mount Sinai Medical School, post-graduate education in health insurance from Health Insurance Associates of America, and post-graduate work in health manpower and facilities, United States Department of Health, Education, and Welfare Training Institute. His professional interests include access and utilization of health and mental health care services by special populations. Dr. Lecca is the author of six books and many government publications. He served as Assistant Commissioner for Mental Health/Mental Retardation/Alcoholism for New York City and was a member of the President's Commission on Mental Health's Task Panel on Special Populations in 1978. He serves on numerous regional and national boards and is a reviewer for several publishers and journals.

DONALD R. BARDILL, Ph.D., is Professor and Dean, School of Social Work, Florida State University, Tallahassee, Florida.

JOSEPH J. BEVILACQUA, Ph.D., is Commissioner, Virginia Department of Mental Health and Mental Retardation, Richmond, Virginia.

LOUIS E. DEMOLL, M.S.W., is Associate Professor, School of Social Work, the University of Texas at Austin, Austin, Texas.

WAYNE H. HOLTZMAN, Ph.D., is President, the Hogg Foundation for Mental Health, the University of Texas at Austin, Austin, Texas.

A. LEVOND JONES, M.S.W., is Manpower Status Coordinator, Division of Human Resource Development, Rhode Island Department of Mental Health, Retardation and Hospitals, Cranston, Rhode Island.

THOMAS J. KANE, D.S.W., is Executive Director, York County Counseling Services, Inc., Saco, Maine.

JOHN S. MCNEIL, D.S.W., is Associate Professor and Director, Community Service Clinic, Graduate School of Social Work, the University of Texas at Arlington, Arlington, Texas.

BENJAMIN E. SAUNDERS is doctoral candidate and Visiting Instructor, School of Social Work, Florida State University, Tallahassee, Florida.

MARK TARAIL, D.S.W., is Director of the Maimonides Community Mental Health Center and of the Department of Community Medicine and Community Health Services, Maimonides Medical Center, Brooklyn, New York.

TED R. WATKINS, D.S.W., is Associate Professor, Department of Sociology, Anthropology, and Social Work, the University of Texas at Arlington, Arlington, Texas.

ROOSEVELT WRIGHT, JR., Ph.D., is Associate Professor and Graduate Advisor, Doctoral Program, Graduate School of Social Work, the University of Texas at Arlington, Arlington, Texas.

PART ONE

Background and Overview

Mental health services currently are being provided to more people in the United States than at any previous time. As the population has increased, so has the number of people needing mental health care. The President's Commission on Mental Health estimated in 1978 that 15 percent of the population needed some form of mental health service. Costs have expanded along with services. Today, over $40 billion is spent annually on mental health services. This section reviews conventional and nontraditional settings in which mental health services are provided and highlights the roles and responsibilities of social workers in this field. In addition, current and future trends in the mental health system are identified. These include an increasing reliance on day hospitals, nursing homes, and outreach programs. It will be shown that state mental hospitals are not necessarily the best place to care for mental patients.

The chapters ahead focus on various trends in the mental health field: the declining role of state mental hospitals, the changing locus of inpatient care, the growth of general hospital psychiatry, the increased use of outpatient mental health facilities, the expansion of nursing home services for mental patients, the rise of community mental health centers, and the growth of the private sector in mental health services. The expanding role of government is documented in an overview of major mental health legislation in the past five decades.

As social workers continue to solidify their position in the mental health field, so must they, along with other mental health professionals, be prepared to respond to changes set in motion by recent trends toward block grants and decentralization of mental health services.

CHAPTER 1

The Convergence of Social Work and Mental Health Services

James W. Callicutt
Pedro J. Lecca

MENTAL DISORDER is a social problem of major proportions (Antonio and Ritzer, 1975, p. 1): an estimated 15 percent of the population need some form of mental health services (President's Commission on Mental Health, 1978), and in 1977 alone roughly two million Americans were admitted to mental facilities as inpatients (U.S. Department of Health and Human Services, 1980).

In discussing the scope of the mental health problem, the President's Commission on Mental Health (1978) noted that "there are large numbers of Americans who suffer from serious emotional problems which are associated with other conditions or circumstances" (p. 8). For example, alcohol abuse represents an annual national cost of over $40 billion. Of the approximately ten million Americans who report recent alcohol related problems, only 10 percent are receiving treatment for alcoholism. Furthermore, problems associated with child abuse, learning disabilities, and physical handicaps may have profound negative consequences for the individual, family, and society. The abuse and misuse of drugs is another area of critical concern in the mental health arena, although services outside the mental health delivery system are often utilized in the treatment of drug and alcohol (also a drug) abuse. In addition, one-third of the six million people who are mentally retarded have multiple handicaps, which often include serious emotional difficulties (President's Commission on Mental Health, 1978). Clearly, the social problem of mental health and mental illness can be neither denied nor ignored.

Social Work: A Key Profession
in the Mental Health Arena

The significance of social work in the field of mental health is underscored by the fact that in 1976 there were 31,212 social worker positions filled in mental health facilities in the United States (National Institute of Mental Health, 1978). These social workers practiced in state and county hospitals, private mental hospitals, Veterans Administration psychiatric services and general hospital psychiatric services, residential treatment centers for emotionally disturbed children, freestanding outpatient clinics, community mental health centers, freestanding day/night facilities, and other multiservice facilities. Additional social workers are found in family and children's agencies, private practice, public schools, and social agencies such as councils on alcoholism and drug abuse.

The professional responsibilities of social workers in the mental health arena are extensive and diverse. Social workers deliver clinical services to clients in all the facilities mentioned. In addition, social workers are engaged in consultation and education, research, and community organization. They also fill planning and administrative positions. For example, Rubin (1979) indicate that "federally funded community mental health centers employ social workers in 33% of their center director positions and 17.5% of their full-time patient care staff positions" (p. 1). Thus, in terms of the sheer number of social workers employed in mental health settings and the importance of their roles, social work is one of the key professions in mental health.

It could be argued further that all social work practice is related to mental health either directly or indirectly. Social work activities in both family service agencies and public assistance agencies bear on the mental health of individuals and families who seek assistance with personal and family problems involving emotional and economic factors. In fact, the provision of at least a minimal financial floor for a troubled individual or family is basic to a client's mental health. However, this book focuses on conventional mental health settings and nontraditional, or emerging, settings that offer explicit mental health services.

The Concept of Mental Health

Thus far we have shown that the social problem of mental health and illness is enormous and that social work is an important profession in the mental health service system. Let us turn now to some of the complex and perplexing definitional problems regarding mental health and social work. As Knee and Lamson (1977) suggested, "Mental health is more subject to description than precise definition. It is one of many human values and is prone to different interpretations and standards that vary with the time, place, culture, and expectations of a social group" (p. 879). Somewhat in this same vein, Schwartz and Schwartz (1968) stated:

> The meaning of the term "mental health" is ambiguous; not only is it difficult to agree on its general application, but even in a single context it may be used in many different ways. This lack of agreement will probably continue because the term has been adopted for a variety of purposes. One conclusion, however, can be reached; "mental health" is not a precise term but an intuitively apprehended idea that is striving for scientific status while also serving as an ideological label. (P. 215)

In further discussing the problem of definition, Schwartz and Schwartz pointed out that

> the word "mental" usually implies something more than the purely cerebral functioning of a person; it also stands for his emotional-affective states, the relationships he establishes with others and a quite general quality that might be called his equilibrium in his sociocultural context. Similarly, "health" refers to more than physical health: it also connotes the individual's intrapsychic balance, the fit of his psychic structure with the external environment and his social functioning. (P. 216)

Freeman and Giovannoni (1969) observed that "the various definitions of mental health can be grouped into three categories: mental health can be considered as a medical, a psychological, or a social phenomenon. The confusion in definition is compounded by the overlapping and merging—unfortunately, there is no integration—of the three positions" (p. 660).

Mead (1963) referred to the notion of "optimum mental health—the fullest, most adequate response that a given individual can make in the particular circumstances in which he finds himself" (p. 7).

The controversy regarding the definitions of mental health and mental illness is far from settled. Szasz (1960) argued that mental illness means nothing more than problems in living. On the other hand, Ausubel (1961), challenging Szasz, insisted that personality disorder is a disease. In common usage the term "mental health" "often means both psychological well-being *and* mental illness" (Schwartz and Schwartz, 1968, p. 216). According to Knee and Lamson (1977), "Mental illness refers to a range of disorders related to an as yet incompletely elucidated complex of physiological, psychological, and sociological factors leading to acute or chronic physical, emotional, and/or behavioral disabilities" (p. 879).

In drawing to a close this discussion of the definitions of mental health and mental illness, let us list the criteria that signal mental health in Jahoda's (1948) treatment of this problem:

1. attitudes of an individual toward his own self
2. growth, development, or self-actualization
3. integration
4. autonomy
5. perception of reality
6. environmental mastery

Barton, a physician, took issue with Jahoda, a psychologist:

> Dr. Jahoda's fundamental position appears to be that the absence of illness and the presence of health overlap but do not coincide. The physician, quite typically I think, works on the basis that they do coincide, for all practical purposes. He sees health as the objective in the prevention, cure or management of disease to the extent that he can help the individual avoid it, recover from it, or compensate for it. (Quoted in Jahoda, 1948, p. 112)

In conclusion, problems in defining mental health and mental illness should not discourage us from struggling with the concepts—to the contrary, they may be enhanced by this exercise.

Definitions of Social Work

There are critical points of intersection between social work and the field of mental health. As Pincus and Minahan (1973) stated:

> Social work is concerned with the interactions between people and their social environment which affect the ability of people to accomplish their life tasks, alleviate distress and realize their aspirations and values. The purpose of social work therefore is to (1) enhance the problem-solving and coping capacities of people, (2) link people with systems that provide them with resources, services, and opportunities, (3) promote the effective and humane operation of these systems, and (4) contribute to the development and improvement of social policy. (P. 9)

Romanyshn (1971) observed that

> social work refers to an occupation and a profession concerned with improving social relationships. It thus has a social service and a social action focus. The field of social welfare may be thought of as encompassing the functions of the various human service professions and occupations: teaching, medicine, psychiatry, clinical psychology, rehabilitation, counseling and so forth. Social work is one of several professions operating within the social welfare network of programs and activities. (P. 54)

Stroup (1960) stated "that social work is the art of bringing various resources to bear on individual, group, and community needs by the application of a scientific method of helping people to help themselves" (pp. 1-2).

Siporin (1975) explicitly referred to the relationship between social work and the resolution of social problems in the following definition: "Social work is defined as a social institutional method of helping people to prevent and resolve their social problems, to restore and enhance their social functioning. Social work is a *social institution,* a human service *profession,* and technical scientific art of *practice"* (p. 3). Gilbert and Specht (1976), looking at the differences between social work and social welfare, pointed out that "the institution of social welfare is much older than the profession of social work." They observed that "the institution serves as a mechanism for mutual support which expresses the collective responsibility of the community for helping its members" (p. 3). They further stated, "In its efforts to provide for mutual support, the institution of social welfare is concerned with the rehabilitation of individuals who have personal problems and with reform of society's need-meeting structures. In practice, social workers are engaged in both rehabilitation and reform activities" (p. 9).

Middleman and Goldberg (1974) claimed that "every instance of social work involves an intervention into the relationship between people and their social environment in order to improve the quality of that relationship. The ultimate target of change may be the people, the social environment, or the relationship itself" (p. 32).

The definitions offered by these authorities clearly suggest the relevance of social work practice in the field of mental health. However, what is not obvious are the roles and functions of social workers in the mental health arena. In the chapters that follow, some of these important activities and functions will be discussed in the context of the major social work methods: direct practice (work with individuals, families, and small groups), community organization, administration, planning, and research. This book takes an institutional perspective, focusing on mental health service settings. Consequently, the important contributions of social workers in family courts, family and children's agencies, and private practice, for example, do not receive specific attention. Moreover, we address social change only indirectly and emphasize mental health rather than mental health and mental retardation (for a current examination of the latter area of social work practice see Dickerson, 1981).

Some Critical Issues in Mental Health Services

The courts have played an important role in the establishment of policies affecting mental health treatment programs. Some judicial decisions have set an agenda of issues that mental health professionals, including social workers, must face. For example, the courts have ruled that patients may not be warehoused in mental hospitals but have a "right to treatment." The "least restrictive institutional alternative" must also be employed.

A strong feeling against involuntary commitment has resulted in "deinstitutionalization" on a large scale. While this policy protects the patient against prolonged and inappropriate confinement, many communities, with inadequate resources, have been unable to cope with the influx of recently discharged patients. (Comptroller General of the United States, 1977). Social workers have been given responsibility for designing and implementing aftercare systems that are reponsive to individual patient needs, while efficiently deploying scarce economic and professional resources.

Prevention often gets lip service; less frequently, this area receives the attention it merits. The development and utilization of creative programs of prevention must be balanced against the service needs of the patient requiring long-term care. A closely related issue is the funding of mental health services. Often, direct care services receive more emphasis than preventive services because of reimbursement policies. This problem demands creativity and commitment on the part of knowledgeable social workers and other mental health professionals faced with diminishing fiscal resources for the human services, including mental health services.

Design and Objectives of the Book

In recognition of the importance of the profession of social work in the expanding array of mental health services, this book focuses on major social work methods within the broad field of mental health. The goal is to serve as a textbook for social work students, as a reference book for social work practitioners, particularly those in the mental health arena, and a resource text in the mental health and social science disciplines. Specifically, this volume embraces seven objectives.

1. To give historical and current information on mental health legislation (and other governmental policies) and services in the United States. The intent is to provide the reader with a base of information to support subsequent chapters and presentations. The provision of mental health services is so directly related to federal, state, and local policies that this background is essential to an understanding of current social work practice in the mental health field.

2. To survey social work practice in mental health settings. Statistical data are given regarding social workers in a range of mental health settings and social worker activities are briefly described to indicate the variety of roles that social workers fill. Historical overviews round out this treatment.

3. To present firsthand accounts by social work practitioners. The chapters on services to individuals, families, and groups; community organization; planning; administration; and research contribute to fulfilling this objective.

4. To provide students and practitioners with new knowledge based on

research and practice experience. The impact of social work on the mental health of individuals and families is of particular interest here.

5. To acquaint the reader with the unique problems of blacks, Hispanics, and Native Americans.

6. To provide an interdisciplinary perspective. Since social workers join with personnel from diverse professions and occupations in delivering services, as well as in planning and administering mental health programs, it is important to appreciate the significance of interdisciplinary approaches and the contributions of psychiatry, clinical psychology, and mental health nursing. Attention is given to the issues of the blurring of professional roles, professional identity, and other costs and benefits associated with an interdisciplinary approach.

7. To identify and forecast trends in the mental health arena, as well as in social work practice as it relates to this arena. Recent innovations include shelters for battered women and children, mutual aid groups, and reliance on natural networks for the prevention of hospitalization and the maintenance in the community of mental health clients.

REFERENCES

ANTONIO, R. J., and RITZER, G. *Social Problems: Values and Interests in Conflict.* Boston: Allyn & Bacon, 1975.

COMPTROLLER GENERAL OF THE UNITED STATES. *Report to the Congress: Returning the Mentally Disabled to the Community: Government Needs to Do More.* U.S. Department of Health, Education, and Welfare and Other Federal Agencies, January 7, 1977.

DICKERSON, M. U., *Social Work Practice with the Mentally Retarded.* New York: Free Press, 1981.

FREEMAN, H. E., and GIOVANNONI, J. M. "Social Psychology of Mental Health." In G. Lindzey and E. Aronson (eds.), *The Handbook of Social Psychology* (2d ed.), vol. 5. Reading, Mass.: Addison-Wesley, 1969.

GILBERT, N., and SPECHT, H. (eds.). *The Emergence of Social Welfare and Social Work.* Itasca, Illinois: F. E. Peacock Publishers, Inc., 1976.

JAHODA, M., *Current Concepts of Positive Mental Health.* New York: Basic Books, 1958.

KNEE, R. T., and LAMSON, W. C. "Mental Health Services." In J. B. Turner (ed.), *Encyclopedia of Social Work* (17th Issue), vol. 2. Washington, D.C.: National Association of Social Workers, 1977.

MEAD, M. "Introduction (Optimum Mental Health)." In A. Deutsch (ed.), *The Encyclopedia of Mental Health,* vol. 1. New York: Watts, 1963.

MIDDLEMAN, R. R., and GOLDBERG, G. *Social Service Delivery: A Structural Approach to Social Work Practice.* New York: Columbia University Press, 1974.

NATIONAL INSTITUTE OF MENTAL HEALTH. *Staffing of Mental Health Facilities, United States, 1976.* Rockville, Md.: U.S. Department of Health, Education, and Welfare, 1978.

PINCUS, A., and MINAHAN, A. *Social Work Practice: Model and Method*. Itasca, Ill.: Peacock, 1973.

PRESIDENT'S COMMISSION ON MENTAL HEALTH. *Report to the President,* vol. 1. Washington D.C.: U.S. Government Printing Office, 1978.

ROMANYSHYN, J. M. *Social Welfare: Charity to Justice*. New York: Random House, 1971.

RUBIN, A. *Community Mental Health in the Social Work Curriculum*. New York: Council on Social Work Education, 1979.

SCHWARTZ, M. S., and SCHWARTZ, C. G. In D. L. Sills (ed.), *International Encyclopedia of the Social Sciences,* vol. 10. New York: Macmillan and Free Press, 1968.

SIPORIN, M. *Introduction to Social Work Practice*. New York: Macmillan, 1975.

STROUP, H. *Social Work* (2d ed.). New York: American, 1960.

U.S. DEPARTMENT OF HEALTH AND HUMAN SERVICES. *Mental Health Statistical Note,* no. 154. Washington, D.C.: 1980.

CHAPTER 2

Current Trends in Mental Health Services and Legislation

Pedro J. Lecca

FOR CENTURIES, mentally ill persons were regarded with a mixture of fear and amusement. They were restrained by chains, beaten, starved, denied medical attention for physical ailments, and even displayed in cages. The mental health system of today reflects a series of both changes in attitude and innovations in technology that began in the United States in the mid-nineteenth century. In 1841, Dorothea Lynde Dix began a crusade for the improvement of the treatment of the insane and other unfortunates housed in jails and almshouses. Her work led to the establishment of state hospitals for the insane in both the United States and Canada (Deutsch, 1949).

Today the mental health field is both very broad and rapidly changing. Whereas mental illness traditionally was viewed as a personal problem or defect, now many mental and emotional disorders are regarded as situational. Accordingly, treatment may involve an entire family. The range of situations implicated in mental dysfunction demands continual innovation in therapy. Practitioners in the field proceed on the premise that people can be helped to cope with the stresses of modern life.

Contemporary Trends in Mental Health Service Delivery

The U.S. mental health system may be described in terms of facilities— Veterans Administration psychiatric hospitals, general hospitals, private clinics, and so on. Table 2.1 shows changes between 1972 and 1978 in the number of beds by facility type, both including and excluding community mental health centers (CMHCs).

Between 1972 and 1978, the U.S. mental health system showed a 36 percent decrease in beds, from 471,800 to 301,011. This decline is best

Table 2.1
Mental Health Beds, by Facility Type, 1972–1978

Mental Health Setting	Year		Percent Change
	1972	1978	
All facility types (excluding CMHCs)	461,191	286,195	−37.9
All facility types (including CMHCs)	471,800	301,011	−36.2
State mental hospitals	361,578	184,079	−49.1
CMHCs	10,609	14,816	+39.7

Source: Department of Health and Human Services, 1981.

understood in the context of other recent developments in the mental health field. These changes in service delivery are reviewed next.

Declining Role of State Mental Hospitals

In 1955, the population of state and county mental hospitals began to decline—a trend that has continued to the present. Between 1955 and 1978, the number of residents fell from an all-time high of 559,000 to 147,283. This decline is related to many factors:

- increased availability and use of alternate care facilities for the aged
- increased availability and use of outpatient and aftercare facilities
- development and use of psychoactive drug treatments
- gradual reduction in the length of stay for admissions
- greater use of community mental health centers and their affiliation with state mental hospitals
- refinement of screening procedures to prevent inappropriate admissions
- changes in state legislation regarding commitment and retention in facilities
- administrative efforts to reduce inpatient populations

While the resident population began diminishing after 1955, the annual number of additions—admissions, readmissions, and returns from leave—to state mental hospitals increased yearly until 1971. Since then, the number of additions has decreased steadily each year, falling 49 percent between 1972 and 1978. The revolving door phenomenon of readmissions to state and county mental hospitals has elicited considerable concern in recent years. While the number of total admissions fell between 1972 and 1978 (in part, because of declining new admissions), the number of readmissions in 1978 was just slightly higher than the 1972 figure.

Changing Locus of Inpatient Care

As the role of the state mental hospital has declined, alternate psychiatric settings, such as general hospital psychiatric units, have taken over inpatient care functions. Greater use of inpatient settings with a more active treatment focus has resulted in a reduction both in the number of days of inpatient care and in the number of psychiatric beds.

If changes in the number of beds in various inpatient facilities are taken as a measure of the shifting locus of care, some interesting patterns can be seen. As Table 2.1 indicates, there was a net decrease in the number of psychiatric beds between 1972 and 1978 for all psychiatric facilities, largely as a result of the drop in the number of state mental hospital beds from 361,578 to 184,079. Despite this net decrease, however, some facilities increased the number of beds during the same period. For example, the number of beds in private psychiatric hospitals rose from 14,412 to 16,637. Even more dramatic, nonfederal general hospital psychiatric units increased their capacity from 23,308 to 29,384 beds.

Growth in General Hospital Psychiatry

There was a marked increase in the number of beds in psychiatric units of nonfederal, short-term general and psychiatric hospitals between 1972 and 1978. This increase contrasted markedly with the decrease in state hospital beds and even exceeded the overall increase for general hospital beds for the same period (American Hospital Association, 1976). The increase in the number of general hospital psychiatric unit beds reflected the creation of many new units.

The overall role of general hospitals in providing mental health services is much larger than figures from their psychiatric facilities suggest. For example, discharges from nonfederal general hospital psychiatric units numbered 516,000 in 1978, whereas discharges with a primary psychiatric diagnosis from all hospital units numbered 1,494,000. In total, 7 percent of the 34 million discharges from nonfederal general hospitals had a diagnosis of mental disorder (National Center for Health Statistics, 1978).

The number of discharges with a secondary but not a primary diagnosis of mental disorder increased 52 percent during the same period (National Center for Health Statistics, 1978). The differential increase in secondary psychiatric diagnoses may reflect the increasing liaison role of psychiatric departments with medical-surgical departments, as well as a continued increase in insurance coverage for mental disorders.

Increased Use of Outpatient Facilities

During the past two decades, mental health care has become increasingly associated with outpatient care. The number of outpatient episodes in organized mental health settings increased from less than 400,000 in 1955 to more than 4.8 million in 1977, a growth far exceeding that experienced by inpatient services. The rate of outpatient episodes per 100,000 population increased from 233 to 2,439 between 1955 and 1978, and outpatient care is now the predominant mode of mental health care. In 1955, 77 percent of the total episodes within organized mental health settings were inpatient; in 1978, the situation was reversed, with 75 percent of the total episodes in outpatient services.

Organized outpatient mental health services may be categorized by their organizational location as follows:

- freestanding outpatient clinics that are not administratively part of, or affiliated with, an inpatient psychiatric facility
- outpatient services affiliated with psychiatric hospitals, both public and private
- outpatient psychiatric services of general hospitals
- outpatient psychiatric services of other mental health facilities, such as residential treatment centers for emotionally disturbed children, outpatient services of federally funded community mental health centers, and clinics of the Veterans Administration

Of the total outpatient mental health services in the United States in January 1978, approximately 10 percent were affiliated with psychiatric hospitals; 17 percent, with general hospitals. Forty-six percent were freestanding psychiatric services; 23 percent were affiliated with federally funded community mental health centers; and 4 percent were affiliated with other types of mental health facilities. Dual affiliation with a general hospital and a community mental health center would put a facility into the CMHC category. Ninety percent of the absolute increase in outpatient admissions between 1972 and 1978 was distributed equally between two types of outpatient settings: freestanding outpatient services and outpatient services of community mental health centers.

Greater Reliance on Nursing Homes

One of the major factors contributing to the decline in the state mental hospital resident population has been the growth of the nursing home industry. Changes in the financing of care occurring in the late 1950s and 1960s enabled the cost of caring for the aged mentally ill person to be shifted from the states to the federal government under Medicare and Medicaid (Chiles, 1975). These financing changes paved the way for nursing homes to flourish and to assume responsibility for long-term care of many chronically mentally ill aged. Between 1954 and 1976, the number of nursing homes increased by about 210 percent, from about 6,500 to 20,185, and the number of nursing home beds grew by almost 730 percent, from 170,000 to 1,407,000.

Between 1969 and 1978, the number of nursing home residents sixty-five years of age and over with a chronic mental disorder increased more than 100 percent, from 96,000 to over 200,000, while the number of residents sixty-five years of age and over in all types of psychiatric hospitals decreased by 49 percent. The net benefit of this trend for the mentally ill elderly has been questioned. Studies of the care provided for these individuals in nursing homes have suggested that reinstitutionalization rather than deinstitutionalization to a less restrictive environment has resulted (Glasscote, 1976). As an example of the impact of financing of care on its locus and quality, this phenomenon has important implications for national health insurance planning.

Growth in Community Mental Health Centers

One aspect of the growth in community based mental health care has been the development of federally funded community mental health centers. The number of community mental health centers increased from 205 in 1969 to 528 in 1975 and to 789 in 1980. As noted earlier, outpatient services at these centers and at freestanding outpatient clinics accounted for 90 percent of the absolute increase in outpatient episodes between 1972 and 1978.

The growth of community mental health centers has resulted in a reorganization of existing facilities and an absolute increase in the number of persons served by organized mental health facilities. CMHCs generally are not newly created but rather are formed by the affiliation of existing community resources—usually general hospital psychiatric services and freestanding outpatient and day treatment programs. In 1978, for example, the 563 CMHCs in operation involved over 2,000 affiliated facilities. General hospital psychiatric services formed a major base for the development of CMHCs, as did state and county operated or supported outpatient services. The state role in the development of CMHCs is demonstrated by the fact that over 30 percent of their funding in 1978 was provided by state governments, equal to the amount provided by the federal government.

In recent years, CMHCs have accounted for the major part of the growth in day treatment services, which were virtually nonexistent twenty years ago.

Between 1972 and 1978, the number of day treatment programs increased dramatically. CMHCs accounted for 233 (50 percent) of the 469 new day treatment programs; freestanding outpatient psychiatric clinics accounted for 168 (36 percent); and general hospitals accounted for 61 (13 percent).

The numerical increase in day treatment programs has been greatest in CMHCs that also sponsor the largest programs, averaging 178 annual admissions per program, versus 79 annual admissions for other settings. Because of this growth, the CMHC day treatment programs now account for more than half of the annual admissions to day treatment services.

Despite dramatic increases in the number of day care programs and admissions to them, day treatment still remains relatively unused in the total spectrum of mental health resources.

Expanded Private Sector Involvement

During the early development of mental health services, public programs were the predominant mode of service delivery. However, this dominance has been eroding at a rapid pace in recent years. The growth in psychiatric services in general hospitals has already been noted. Similarly, private psychiatric hospitals have grown in number from 151 in 1968 to over 190 in 1978 and have assumed an increasing role in inpatient care.

While national data are not available, there has probably been a significant increase in the number of people under the care of private practitioners (Redlich and Kellert, 1978). The number of people seen privately in psychiatrists' and psychologists' offices has been estimated at almost 1.3 million, or 20 percent of the total number of people seen in 1975 in the specialty mental health sector (Regier, 1978). Indeed, the population seen in all private settings—hospitals, clinics, and offices—probably represents about half the people receiving organized mental health services.

Development of the Mental Health System through Legislation: Initial Federal Involvement

At the turn of the century, overcrowded and understaffed state hospitals were the primary facility for the care of the mentally ill. Local and state authorities controlled these institutions and there were no federal activities related to mental illness until the early 1900s (Ridenour, 1961).

One of the first federal initiatives in mental health was the examination of potential immigrants (Grand, 1968). The high incidence of first admissions of foreign-born persons to New York State mental hospitals in the opening decades of the twentieth century helped to develop public recognition of mental disorders as a national health problem (Grand, 1968). Important developments at the turn of the century included the opening of psychiatric wards in general hospitals, the establishment of social work programs in psychiatric care, the beginning of some outpatient and aftercare services, and the establishment in a few cities of psychopathic hospitals for diagnosis and preliminary care of patients to avert long-term, custodial care.

Involvement of the federal government in mental health services began in a limited way in 1930, when the Public Health Service established the Division of Mental Hygiene, which in 1949 became the National Institute of Mental Health.

From their inception to the mid-twentieth century, state asylums and mental institutions continued to care for the mentally ill through the provision of custodial services and the use of isolation. Modern state hospital licensure laws were enacted after 1946 and were applied to private mental facilities, generally exempting state mental hospitals. In 1948, the American Psychiatric Association established an inspection rating system for mental hospitals, and in 1958 the Joint Commission on Accreditation of Hospitals began to inspect and accredit mental hospitals and general hospitals (Roemer, 1975).

The first major mental health law in the United States was enacted in 1946, the National Mental Health Act.

National Mental Health Act of 1946 (P.L. 79–487)

MAJOR EMPHASIS. Improve the mental health of people in the United States by promoting investigations, experiments, and demonstration projects related to the cause, diagnosis, and treatment of psychiatric disorders.

World War II, by revealing extremely large numbers of mentally disturbed men, led to extensive federal involvement in mental health services. The war was hardly over when the National Mental Health Act of 1946 propelled the government into a position of prominence in the mental health field (Roemer, 1975).

The war had created wide awareness of the high cost of mental illness and the potential effectiveness of psychiatric care. As a result of this changed background of public knowledge and opinion, the National Mental Health Act of 1946 was passed by Congress. The act provided for (1) funding of research on the cause, diagnosis, and treatment of psychiatric disorders; (2) training of professional personnel; and (3) assistance to the states in the creation of pilot and demonstration studies for prevention, diagnosis, and treatment. From this major federal legislation there emerged the wide-ranging programs of the National Institute of Mental Health (Grand, 1965).

Despite passage of the National Mental Health Act in 1946, the federal government had no direct authority to provide and maintain clinics and other treatment services throughout the country until the establishment in

1949 of the National Institute of Mental Health (NIMH). The Community Services Branch of NIMH offered consultant services, field demonstrations, and grants-in-aid to assist state programs. Until 1965 NIMH was unique among the National Institutes of Health in sponsoring service activities (Grand, 1965).

The founders of NIMH were Public Health Service officers with backgrounds in psychiatry. They considered the institute's primary function to be the support of the study of mental illness, and they tended to define the field of mental health very narrowly. Their conception of the mental health system did not give high priority to the prevention of mental illness (Duhl and Leopold, 1968), although the National Mental Health Act had been broadly conceived not only to combat mental illness but also to promote mental health. The comprehensiveness of the act nevertheless had important implications for the development of the field.

Mental Health Study Act of 1955 (P.L. 84-182)

MAJOR EMPHASIS.   Provide for an objective, thorough, and nationwide analysis and reevaluation of the human and economic problems of mental illness.

The publication in 1910 of Abraham Flexner's findings on medical education heralded a rapid and radical improvement in the teaching and practice of medicine in the United States (1910). He concluded that medical education was fragmented, lacked standards, and was ineffective in preparing students for medical practice. Approximately forty years later, in 1953, Kenneth Appel, then president of the American Psychiatric Association, appealed for a survey that would produce for mental health the kind of results that had come out of the Flexner Report. Through the vigorous efforts of Appel, his medical colleagues, and other interested individuals and groups, the Joint Commission on Mental Illness and Health was established in 1955 to study the problems of mental and emotional illness (Connery, 1968). Simultaneously, Congress passed the Mental Health Study Act of 1955. Funds were authorized for a total of $1,250,000 for organizations to carry out research on diagnosing, caring for, and rehabilitating the mentally ill. The newly organized Joint Commission on Mental Illness and Health was selected to undertake the intensive investigation the act sought to encourage.

The commission's report listed four major barriers to developing mental health programs: (1) the negative attitude of the public, (2) insufficient professional personnel, (3) continuation of custodial care hospitals, and (4) lack of effective long-term research (Joint Commission, 1961). The recommendations called for increased recruitment of professional personnel, as well as the training of paraprofessionals; establishment of full-time mental health clinics; provision of short-term hospitalization in general hospitals; establishment of intensive psychiatric treatment centers; and creation of aftercare and rehabilitation services. The report favored direct federal support for services, with sharing of financial responsibilities by state and local units, and increased local responsibility in developing services and providing financial support (Nacman, 1977).

The final report of the Joint Commission on Mental Illness and Health (1961), *Action for Mental Health,* provided the background for the historic special message of President Kennedy to the Congress early in 1963. This message, in turn, gave impetus to the development of the community mental health centers program.

Community Mental Health Centers Construction Act of 1963 (P.L. 88–164)

MAJOR EMPHASIS.   Improve mental health through grants for construction of community mental health centers.

President Kennedy's 1963 message on mental health set the stage for the Community Mental Health Centers Construction Act. This legislation mandated essential services, identifying consultation and education services as methods of prevention. Thus, a public policy of prevention was established that would influence other programs.

The final report of the Joint Commission on Mental Illness and Health opened an era of unprecedented federal action in the care of the mentally ill. Some community oriented mental health professionals believed that the commission was concerned mainly with mental illness and that the report was hospital oriented (Grand, 1968). Therefore, in response to the commission's report, these professionals emphasized the need for community mental health centers to provide a comprehensive network of mental health activities at the local level.

The Community Mental Health Centers Construction Act of 1963 represented a compromise between the hospital orientation of the commission's report and the comprehensive community program urged by community oriented professional and lay persons interested in mental health (Duhl and Leopold, 1968). This law, which made grants available for the construction of research centers and community health centers, espoused two principal objectives: to provide comprehensive mental health services and to provide adequate services for clients unable to pay. The law also spelled out the comprehensive services to be provided: inpatient and outpatient care; partial hospitalization; twenty-four-hour emergency services; consultation and education; diagnostic services; rehabilitative services; precare and aftercare services in the community; and training, research, and evaluation.

Centers were to be organized in conformity with a state plan, with planning and coordination vested in an advisory council composed of representatives from nongovernmental and state agencies, as well as consumers of services. Services were to be provided to all residents of a designated geographic area; the law established no minimal residence requirements. Amendments to the act in 1965, 1967, and 1970 authorized additional financial assistance for staffing, expansion, and renovation of the community mental health centers.

The Community Mental Health Centers Construction Act of 1963 and its 1975 amendment (P.L. 94-63) represented an enormous outpouring of federal funds into the area of mental health, and many services were being provided. Perhaps the greatest contribution of this legislation was the impetus it gave to the deinstitutionalization of the mentally ill (Mechanic, 1979). However, planning on a national scale was needed to provide overall guidance in the development, financing, distribution, utilization, and evaluation of mental health and health services. In the early 1970s, Congress once again attempted to meet the nation's need for comprehensive health care. The National Health Planning and Resources Development Act was passed by Congress in 1974 and signed into law by President Ford on January 4, 1975.

National Health Planning and Resources Development Act of 1975 (P.L. 93-641)

MAJOR EMPHASIS.   Amend the Public Health Service Act to insure the development of a national health policy and of effective state and area health planning and resource development programs.

Often referred to as the most significant health legislation in the last decade, this law was viewed by many as a necessary forerunner to national health insurance. The assumption is that through P.L. 93-641 the health care delivery system can be made sufficiently efficient to meet the demands that national health insurance will place on it.

The National Health Planning and Resources Development Act identified many national issues requiring attention, including the need to provide equal access to quality health care at a reasonable cost, inflationary increases brought about by the infusion of large federal sums into the health care system via Medicaid and Medicare, lack of uniformly effective methods of delivering health care, poor distribution of services, greater emphasis on the more costly services of hospital care rather than on less expensive and more appropriate alternative medical services, failure to involve the provider of health services in the planning and improvement of health care services, and inadequate efforts made to educate the public in personal health care and the availability of services (Hyman, 1976).

In recognition of the magnitude of the problems and the urgency of their solution, the act proposed to facilitate the development of recommendations for a national health planning policy; to augment areawide and state planning for health services, manpower, and facilities; and to authorize financial assistance for the development of resources to further these goals. Additionally, the act authorized the issuance of national guidelines for health planning by the secretary of health, education, and welfare and established national health priorities.

This act used the term "health" in a generic sense, and mental health was not singled out for particular attention. However, the intent of Congress that the term "health" be considered comprehensively was clear from the explicit inclusion of the Community Mental Health Centers Construction Act in regard to required review and approval of both individual mental health projects and state mental health plans by the health agencies (Kelty, 1978).

The National Health Planning and Resources Development Act was far more ambitious and complex than any other health planning law. The extent to which effective planning for mental health will be accomplished through implementation of the act is still to be determined. It was only after long discussions with local, state, and federal agencies that mental health professionals accepted the review and approval process mandated by the act; mental health professionals object also to the secondary role accorded mental health services. The next few months will be critical for P.L. 93–641 in merging physical and mental health within a national planning strategy. Continuation of this legislation is problematic. If this act is not continued, then many of the planning initiatives already established will fall by the wayside.

Relationship between P.L. 93–641 and P.L. 94–63

P.L. 93–641 and 94–63 (the 1975 amendment to the Community Mental Health Centers Construction Act), passed within a few months of each other, mandated specific planning and resource development responsibilities—the former for health systems agencies (HSAs), state health planning and development agencies (SHPDAs), and statewide health coordinating councils (SHCCs); the latter for state mental health authorities (SMHAs). The considerable overlap between the two laws created problems for, and tensions between, mental health and health planners. As regulations and legislative amendments are proposed that tie together mental health and

health planning, attention has come to be focused on who has what pre-
rogatives.

Community Support Projects

PL 94-63, as amended in 1977, with state cooperation promoted community or statewide demonstration projects for adult chronically mentally ill
patients. It also served to prepare deinstitutionalized patients for relocation
into the community. This initiative was to stimulate and promote group
housing, halfway housing with modalities of job training, independent living skills, and other psychosocial components.

Originally in 1977, funding was provided for Washington, D.C., and
eighteen states: New Jersey, New York, Montana, Colorado, Georgia, Min-
nesota, Alabama, Florida, Oregon, Arizona, Missouri, South Dakota,
Massachusetts, California, Maine, Maryland, Michigan, and Texas. This
federal initiative has contributed to the development of diverse community
support systems throughout the country. For FY '82 4.8 million dollars was
appropriated to fund existing programs and twenty additional projects at
the $120,000 level. It is anticipated by the federal government that the states
will continue these projects, possibly out of block grants resources.

Community Mental Health Centers and Biomedical
Research Extension Act of 1978 (P.L. 95-622)

MAJOR EMPHASIS. Amend the Community Mental Health Centers Construction Act to continue funding authorization for planning, operation
grants, and services.

A two-year extension of the community mental health centers program
was approved, authorizing for fiscal years 1979 and 1980, respectively, $1.5
million and $1 million for planning grants; $34.5 million and $35 million
for initial operation grants; $20 million and $3 million for consultation and
education services grants; $30 million and $25 million for conversion grants;
$8 million and $9 million for the rape prevention and control program; and
$25 million for fiscal year 1979, with no funding for fiscal year 1980, for
financial distress grants. Other provisions allow a CMHC to use grant funds
in the year following the year in which they are given if they are not obli-
gated during the grant year. Moreover, up to 1 percent of appropriations
can be used for evaluating activities of community mental health centers.

Newly added provisions permit centers to phase in required services.
Under the previous legislation, centers had to provide inpatient, emergency,
and outpatient services; assistance to courts and other public agencies in

screening clients to determine whether inpatient treatment or treatment through the center was appropriate; follow-up care for individuals discharged from inpatient facilities; and consultation and education services, including activities designed to develop effective mental health programs, coordination of the delivery of mental health services, and activities that otherwise would increase public awareness of mental health problems. In the second stage, the phase-in of services, CMHCs are to provide day treatment and other partial hospitalization services, specialized services for children, specialized services for the elderly, halfway house services, and alcoholism and drug addiction programs if these are needed. A center must either offer this second group of services upon its establishment or have a plan for the provision of these services within three years. Inpatient, emergency, and halfway house services can be provided through appropriate arrangements with health professionals and others serving the residents of the catchment area.

A separate mental health authority has been established under the general Public Health Services Act authority for grants for comprehensive health planning and public health services. Under this new provision, the secretary of health and human services can make grants to state mental health authorities to assist them in meeting the costs of carrying out their functions under the health planning law and the community mental health centers program, as well as in meeting the costs of providing mental health services. Requirements for federal support relate to insuring the appropriateness of services provided; the appropriate use of federal funds, including necessary fiscal controls; and the carrying out of a program by the state mental health authority that will prescribe and enforce minimal standards relating to the care and treatment of individuals with mental health problems. Allocation of funds among the states is made on the basis of population and financial need. The law authorizes $15 million, $20 million, and $25 million for fiscal years 1979–1981, respectively, for these state mental health grants.

Mental Health Systems Act of 1980 (P.L. 96-398)

MAJOR EMPHASIS.   Provide grants for community mental health centers and special population groups, for prevention programs, promotion of mental health, and extension of Community Mental Health Centers Construction Act.

This act preserved some mental health components of earlier legislation and included provisions to make mental health services more accessible and effective for the general population and, in particular, for special groups. The Mental Health Systems Act provided within the National Institute of

Mental Health for a National Institute of Mental Health prevention unit, an associate director for minority concerns, grants for protection and advocacy programs for the mentally ill, grants for rape prevention and control, grants for services to rape victims, a one-year extension of the Community Mental Health Centers Act, and a report on basic living needs of chronically mentally ill individuals.

In the 1980s federal funding for mental health programs will be through block grants through the states. In many states this will mean cutbacks in the mental health delivery system, as well as consolidation of programs.

Utilization and Staffing of Mental Health Facilities

During the year 1975, an estimated 15 percent of the U.S. population needed mental health services (Regier, Goldberg, and Taube, 1978). Of this group 15 percent were receiving care from the specialty mental health sector; 3.4 percent from general hospital inpatient and nursing home sector; 6 percent from both specialty mental health sectors and primary care-outpatient medical sector (overlap); 54.1 percent from the primary care-outpatient medical sector; and 21.5 percent were either receiving some assistance or services from other service sectors or not receiving services at all.

Unfortunately, data are not available to differentiate among the number of persons with mental disorders who receive no health or mental health treatment, those who may be in correctional institutions, and those who are served by family service agencies, religious counselors, and other social welfare agencies outside the usually defined health arena. This is a critical area for research. There are considerable differences in the diagnostic characteristics of patients seen in these various settings. For example, patients who come to nonpsychiatric physicians are more likely to present problems associated with anxiety and depression, personality disorders, and psychophysiologic disturbance. Persons with more severe disorders, such as schizophrenia, major affective disorders, organic brain syndromes, and other conditions requiring intensive specialized therapies are more likely to receive inpatient treatment in the mental health sector. Persons using outpatient services in the mental health sector present a broader spectrum of mental disorders, with variations reflecting the admission policies of the clinic, its relationship to the mental hospitals serving the community, and referral practices of physicians, local public health, and social agencies.

As noted earlier, the 1970s saw a dramatic drop in the patient population of state mental hospitals. The number of residents at the end of 1978 (147,283) was 49 percent of the number at the end of 1955 (558,922), the year in which the mental hospital population was at its highest level.

Federally Funded Community Mental Health Centers

Past and recent legislation has been an important aspect of the growth in community based mental health care. The number of community mental health centers increased from 205 in 1969 to 528 in 1975 and to 789 in 1980. Previously, I pointed out that the outpatient services of these centers and of freestanding outpatient clinics accounted for 90 percent of the absolute increase in outpatient episodes between 1972 and 1978. The proliferation of community mental health centers has resulted in a reorganization of existing facilities and an increase in the number of persons served by organized mental health facilities.

Social Workers in Mental Health Settings

At the mental health facilities included in Table 2.2, most social work positions at the master's level and above were found in community mental health centers (26.9 percent of the total) and freestanding outpatient clinics (24.4 percent). In both settings, full-time equivalent social work positions outnumbered those for psychiatry and psychology, constituting almost half the total positions held by these three provider groups. Although the number involved was smaller, social workers were also predominant among these provider types in residential treatment centers and freestanding day/night facilities and other multiservice facilities. In state and county mental hospitals, general hospitals, and private mental hospitals, the number of psy-

Table 2.2
Practice Settings of Social Workers in Mental Health, 1976

Mental Health Setting	Full-time Equivalent Positions	
	Number	Percent
Community mental health centers	5,106	26.9
Freestanding outpatient clinics	4,630	24.4
State and county mental hospitals	3,181	16.8
Psychiatric units of general hospitals	2,072	10.9
Veterans Administration psychiatric facilities	1,348	7.1
Private mental hospitals	652	3.4
Residential treatment centers	1,410	7.4
Freestanding day/night facilities and other multiservice facilities	582	3.1
Total	18,981	100.0

Source: Rosenstein and Taube, 1978.

chiatrists' positions surpassed that of social workers, while the number of social worker positions exceeded that for psychologists. It might be hypothesized that the involvement of social workers in psychiatric services like evaluation and psychotherapy is greater in settings that have fewer paraprofessional provider types (e.g., outpatient clinics and community mental health centers). In hospital settings, where psychiatrists are plentiful, the social worker may be more involved with the traditional social work functions of casework and service integration (National Center for Health Services Research, 1977).

Trends and Issues

As a result of the development of community based programs for the diagnosis, treatment, and rehabilitation of persons with mental disorders, the locus of care has shifted from the large state mental hospitals to community based facilities, particularly to outpatient services and community mental health centers. To illustrate, in 1955, 1.7 million episodes of care were handled by the universe of facilities that report to the National Institute of Mental Health. Of these, 49 percent were handled by state and county mental hospitals; 23 percent, by outpatient psychiatric services; 16 percent, by general hospital inpatient psychiatric units; and 12 percent, by all other facilities. By 1978, the number of episodes of care reported by all facilities had increased to over 7 million. Of these, 9 percent were reported by state and county mental hospitals; 47 percent, by outpatient psychiatric services; 29 percent, by community mental health centers; 9 percent, by general hospital inpatient psychiatric units; and 6 percent, by other reporting facilities.

These changes have had a marked effect on the composition of the institutional population. In 1950, 1.6 million persons (1 percent of the population of the United States) were in institutions. The largest group was in mental institutions (39 percent); the second largest, in homes for the aged and dependent (19 percent); and the third largest, in correctional institutions (17 percent). In 1978, the number of persons in institutions amounted to over 2.4 million, about 1.2 percent of the total population. The largest portion was in homes for the aged and dependent (44 percent); the next largest, in mental institutions (20 percent); and the third largest, in correctional institutions (15 percent).

The changes in the numbers of persons in specific types of institutions have been the result of a variety of factors such as social legislation, new discoveries for treatment of disorders, demographic changes, increasing costs of general hospital and domiciliary care for persons with chronic illnesses, shifting social conditions and problems, racist and other discriminatory practices, and inadequate community programs and inappropriate living arrangements for persons who are aged, disabled, or mentally ill. Some general factors (Alcohol, Drug Abuse, and Mental Health Administration, 1976) and issues of particular importance to social workers concerned with mental health planning and policy development deserve mention:

1. About 15 percent of Americans are estimated to have mental disorders within any one-year period.
2. Most receive care from a variety of sources, but primarily from the general health not the specialty mental health service system.
3. As many as 22 percent of those with mental disorders may receive no diagnostic assessment or treatment.
4. The specialty mental health service system, once largely geared toward long-term inpatient care in public facilities, is becoming increasingly oriented toward short-term and outpatient care in the private sector.
5. The length of stay in specialty mental health inpatient facilities has descreased appreciably, as has the number of inpatient beds.
6. The locus of inpatient care of the mentally ill is shifting from state and county mental hospitals to several other settings, particularly nursing homes and psychiatric inpatient units of general hospitals.
7. The diagnoses that bring people to mental health services are primarily schizophrenia and depression, although the major diagnoses vary considerably by setting, with a predominance of less severe disorders in outpatient settings.
8. The growth of community mental health centers has provided new service resources and has had a profound effect on outpatient care—particularly day treatment—but has not yet achieved its full potential in creating a more equitable geographic distribution of services and personnel.
9. The distribution of patients among various types of mental health facilities is related to many factors, including diagnosis, income level, age, cultural and racial background, and health insurance coverage. There are still many barriers that restrict freedom of choice for some individuals (particularly those with low incomes and no insurance), and these may result in a less than optimal match of patients and services.
10. Various racial and cultural minority groups are unevenly represented in the range of mental health service settings. Although the admission rates of minority group members are increasing in several settings that were previously little utilized, such as the psychiatric units of general hospitals and private psychiatric hospitals, large differences in admission rates still exist.
11. Mental health personnel, like mental health facilities, are unevenly distributed geographically, with rural areas notably lacking in mental health services.

The scope and quality of mental health care available to the American people in the future will depend on policy decisions at all levels of government and on the kind and degree of participation by the public and the private sector in organizing and financing mental health services. The structure and level of funding for mental health services in the United States in the 1980s will depend most notably on the implementation of block grant legislation.

REFERENCES

ALCOHOL, DRUG ABUSE, and MENTAL HEALTH ADMINISTRATION, LEGISLATIVE SERVICES UNIT. "Current Status of State Community Mental Health Services Legislation." Rockville, Md.: The Administration, 1976.

AMERICAN HOSPITAL ASSOCIATION. *Hospital Statistics, 1976.* Chicago: American Hospital Association, 1976.

————. *Guide to the Health Care Field and Hospital Statistics.* Chicago: American Hospital Association, 1976.

BABIGIAN, H. M. "The Impact of Community Mental Health Centers on the Utilization of Services." *Archives of General Psychiatry* 1977, *34*(4):385-394.

BOURNE, P. G. *"Psychological Aspects of Combat."* Paper given at the Symposium on Stress, Department of Psychiatry, University of Virginia, June 1969.

CAPLAN, R. *Psychiatry and the Community in Nineteenth-Century America.* New York: Basic Books, 1969.

CHILES, C. L. *A Study of the Failure to Implement Alternate Care Recommendations for Patients in Mental Hospitals and Nursing Homes.* U.S. Department of Commerce, National Technical Information Service, December 1975.

CONNERY, R. H. *The Politics of Mental Health.* New York: Columbia University Press, 1968.

DEPARTMENT OF HEALTH and HUMAN SERVICES. "Mental Health Statistical Note No. 155." Rockville, Md.: Alcohol, Drug Abuse, and Mental Health Administration, 1981.

DEUTSCH, A. *The Mentally Ill in America.* New York: Columbia University Press, 1949.

DUHL, L. F., and LEOPOLD, R. L. *Mental Health and Urban Social Policy.* San Francisco: Jossey-Bass, 1968.

FLEXNER, A. *Medical Education in the United States and Canada.* A Report to the Carnegie Foundation for the Advancement of Teaching. Carnegie Foundation Bulletin no 4. New York: 1910.

GLASSCOTE, R., BEIGEL, A., BUTTERFIELD, A., JR., and CLARK, E. *Old Folks at Home.* Washington, D.C.: American Psychiatric Association, 1976.

GRAND, J. L. "The United States: A Historical Perspective." In R. H. Williams and L. D. Ozarin (eds.), *Community Mental Health.* San Francisco: Jossey-Bass, 1968.

HYMAN, H. H. *Health Planning.* Germantown, Md.: Aspen, 1976.

JOINT COMMISSION ON MENTAL ILLNESS AND HEALTH. *Action for Mental Health.* New York: Science Editions, 1961.

KELTY, E. J. "Mental Health in Health Planning: Fitting Square Programs into Round Holes." *American Journal of Health Planning* 1978, *3*:65–70.

MECHANIC, D. *Future Issues in Health Care: Social Policy and the Rationing of Medical Services.* New York: Free Press, 1979.

NACMAN, M. "Social Workers in Mental Health Services." In *Encyclopedia of Social Work* (17th Issue). Washington, D.C.: National Association of Social Workers, 1977, pp. 897–904.

NATIONAL CENTER FOR HEALTH SERVICES RESEARCH. *Health Resources Statistics, 1976–1977.* Washington, D.C.: U.S. Government Printing Office, 1977.

NATIONAL CENTER FOR HEALTH STATISTICS. *Inpatient Utilization of Short-Stay Hospitals by Diagnosis, United States, 1975.* Washington, D.C.: U.S. Government Printing Office, 1978.

REDLICH, F., and KELLERT, S. R. "Trends in American Mental Health." *American Journal of Psychiatry* 1978, *135*(1):22–28.

REGIER, D. A., GOLBERG, I. D., and TAUBE, C. A. "The De Facto U.S. Mental Health Service System: A Public Health Perspective." Manuscript, Division of Biometry and Epidemiology, National Institute of Mental Health, 1978.

———. "The De Facto U.S. Mental Health Services System." *Archives of General Psychiatry* 1978, *35*(6):685–693.

RIDENOUR, N. *Mental Health in the United States: A Fifty-Year History.* Cambridge: Harvard University Press, 1961.

ROEMER, R., KRAMER, C., and FRINK, J. E. *Planning Urban Health Services.* New York: Springer, 1975.

ROSENSTEIN, M. J., and TAUBE, C. A. *Staffing of Mental Health Facilities, United States, 1976.* Rockville, Md.: National Institute of Mental Health, 1978.

CHAPTER 3

Contemporary Settings and the Rise of the Profession in Mental Health

James W. Callicutt

SOCIAL WORKERS TODAY practice in a wide range of mental health settings. This chapter traces the beginnings of social work practice and professional education, focusing on mental health from the early 1900s. Then prominent social worker roles and activities relative to these major practice environments are reviewed. I also discuss the interacting influences of the child guidance movement, the world wars, the community mental health movement, and various governmental policies. Last, predictions are made regarding future trends in social work practice in the mental health arena.

Social work, one of the four core disciplines in the field of mental health, makes a major contribution to the professional staffing of mental health facilities in the United States. In January 1978, for example, the 28,073 full-time equivalent social work positions almost equaled the combined number of psychiatrists (14,450) and psychologists (16,458) (National Institute of Mental Health, 1980). Furthermore, except for nurses, the fourth and remaining mental health core discipline, social workers are the largest professional group staffing mental health facilities.

Data for 1972, 1974, 1976, and 1978 clearly show marked increases in the number of full-time equivalent professional positions, including social work, in mental health facilities in the United States (National Institute of Mental Health, 1978, 1980). However, with the current shifting of governmental responsibilities in the mental health arena and the accompanying unsettled climate regarding the role of the federal government in developing mental health policy initiatives, it is not appropriate to make projections for the future based on these trend data.

The Evolution of the Profession

Practice

The creation in 1905 of the social work program by Dr. Richard Cabot and Ida Cannon at Massachusetts General Hospital "might be considered a beginning point" (Nacman, 1977, p. 899) in social work's involvement in mental health. Dr. James J. Putnam, chief of neurological services at Massachusetts General, was extremely interested in this new social service department. In 1906 he appointed a full-time assistant, Edith N. Burleigh, an experienced social worker, to whom he gave special training (Cannon, 1923; Southard and Jarrett, 1922). Jointly they developed principles derived from the interrelation of medicine and social work and applied them in understanding and treating mentally ill patients. Margherita Ryther, Burleigh's successor, identified three main service categories: (1) social investigation before making plans for disposition and treatment, (2) social investigation as a contribution to diagnosis, and (3) social study to supplement the physician's treatment (Cannon, 1923). Although somewhat different terminology may now be employed, these services are still performed by the social worker in many mental health settings.

Shortly after the initiation of the program at Massachusetts General, Bellevue Hospital and Cornell Clinic developed programs in New York (Nacman, 1977). Similar programs were established in other states during these years.

In 1906 the first aftercare agent, E. H. Horton, a graduate of the New York School of Philanthropy, was hired by the New York Charities Aid Association (Deutsch, 1949; French, 1940). Horton was assigned to two hospitals to demonstrate the value of providing social services to patients who were well enough to leave the hospital but who needed help in locating a place to live, an appropriate job, and community resources (Woodward, 1960). So successful was the demonstration that legislation was enacted in 1913 to allow for the development of similar services in all mental hospitals in New York State. Meeting the needs of patients returning to the community continues to be a major function of social workers in the mental health service delivery system.

The term "psychiatric social worker" was first applied to social workers in mental hospitals in 1913. Mary C. Jarrett, a pioneer in this field, was responsible for assigning this title to social work staff at the newly opened Boston Psychopathic Hospital (Woodward, 1960). She "conceived of the work as an independent service in strict accordance with the physician's plans but with special activities not directed by him" (French, 1940, p. 37). The social service department at Boston Psychopathic Hospital was organized around four functional categories: casework services, executive duties (efficient management of the outpatient clinic), public education, and research.

In 1918 Massachusetts again broke new ground. The state established a Division of Social Service responsible for coordinating and planning social services at the state mental hospitals (Stroup, 1960). This was the first attempt to coordinate psychiatric social work on a state level.

Education

Jarrett, at Boston Psychopathic Hospital, accepted students from Simmons College School of Social Work for field placements in 1914 (Ferguson, 1969). She, Dr. E. E. Southard, the hospital's director, and others also gave courses in psychiatry and psychiatric social work at Simmons (French, 1940). Thus, we see the initiation of special training for psychiatric social workers.

The same decade saw the opening of Phipps Clinic at Johns Hopkins Hospital in Baltimore (French, 1940). Dr. Adolf Meyer, the clinic's director, had been active in planning aftercare for patients in New York. Meyer brought to Phipps Clinic a keen interest in social service that was tied to his holistic approach to mental disease. In 1913 Meyer appointed the first social worker to the clinic staff. This service later developed a program that would maintain close relationships with the schools and community social agencies relative to the care of children. The clinic also participated in the training of social work students from the School of Economics at Johns Hopkins University.

The Training School for Psychiatric Social Work opened at Smith College several years later (Deutsch, 1949). On another front, as part of the Commonwealth Fund program for the prevention of delinquency, the New York School of Social Work established the Bureau of Children's Guidance in 1921 (Lee and Kenworthy, 1930). The bureau "was to prepare students for psychiatric social work as practiced in child guidance clinics and in other psychiatric agencies and to give students preparing for other fields of social work a working knowledge of social psychiatry" (Lee and Kenworthy, 1930, p. 157).

Having briefly discussed the auspicious beginnings of professional education for psychiatric social workers, let us now look at other forces related to the mental health focus in social work practice and education.

The Child Guidance Movement

A project to set up demonstration child guidance clinics throughout the country was financed in the 1920s by the Commonwealth Fund (Stroup, 1960). The National Committee for Mental Hygiene, on behalf of the Commonwealth Fund, selected St. Louis as the site of its first child guidance clinic, which opened in 1922 (Stevenson, 1934). Eventually, seven more clinics were set up. The professional staff of the St. Louis clinic included a psychiatrist, a psychologist, and a psychiatric social worker. This team pattern continues to be used in child guidance and mental health clinics.

Many professionals were skeptical about the addition of service to the emotionally disturbed child, thinking that their domain was being invaded. Although "social work was among the disciplines that did not welcome the development of child guidance clinics, . . . [it] was the [psychiatric] social worker on the treatment team that eventually managed to influence the direction of child guidance services" (Goldsmith, 1977, p. 894). This movement was in the direction of social or community psychiatry.

Social Workers in the Military Service

World War I increased both the incidence of psychiatric problems and the need for the treatment of military and civilian personnel. Recognition of this increased need for psychiatric social workers encouraged the initiation of the formal training program at what is now the Smith College School for Social Work. Social services were organized for federal hospitals by the American Red Cross at the request of the U.S. surgeon general in 1919 (French, 1940).

During World War II, enlisted men were first assigned as social workers to a neuropsychiatric team at the mental hygiene service at Fort Monmouth, New Jersey (Rooney, 1965). In 1943 the position classification "social work technician" was established by the Army, officially recognizing the value of the military psychiatric social worker. Several years later, an officer level occupational specialty classification, "psychiatric social worker," was introduced.

According to testimony by the director of the Selective Service System, over a million draft registrants had been rejected for military service by August 1, 1945, because of neuropsychiatric disorders (Deutsch, 1949). William C. Menninger elaborated: "During the period of January 1, 1942 through December 30, 1945 . . . there were approximately one million patients with neuropsychiatric disorders admitted to army hospitals. This represented a rate of 45 admissions per 1,000 troops per year and constituted 6 percent of all admissions" (quoted in Deutsch, 1949, p. 467). Deutsch also quoted Captain Francis J. Braceland's review of wartime psychiatry in the U.S. Navy:

> In the U.S. Navy from January 1, 1942, to July 1, 1945, a period which roughly covers the war years, there were 149,281 patients admitted to various naval hospitals and dispensaries throughout the world for all reasons which could be subsumed under the heading of psychiatric diseases. This comprehensive category

includes everything from mild emotional instability to malignant schizophrenia. Of this number of patients, 76,721 individuals had to be separated from the naval service, and this figure represents roughly 32.4 percent of the total naval medical separations during the entire war. (P. 467)

Post-World War II Federal Government Influences

In order to train personnel for the new facilities needed to provide mental hospital care for large numbers of veterans, the Veterans Administration, together with the Menninger Clinic, launched a major program (Ferguson, 1969). At about the same time, Congress passed the National Mental Health Act, and in 1949 the National Institute of Mental Health (NIMH) was established. NIMH has played a major role in supporting the professional education of mental health personnel. As part of this effort, schools of social work have been encouraged to train personnel specifically in the area of mental health.

The Social Work Education Branch of the National Institute of Mental Health provides grants to graduate schools of social work, thereby supporting the operation of specialized mental health educational programs. These grants include support for trainees. While support was broadly targeted initially, NIMH recently has outlined training priorities. Criteria reflecting these priorities are used when training grant applications are evaluated for potential funding. However, continued funding for these projects is threatened and uncertain.

Accredited Social Work Education Programs

In 1981 there were 303 baccalaureate and 87 master's degree programs in the United States accredited by the Council on Social Work Education (Rubin, 1982). There were 43 doctoral programs; however, doctoral programs are not accredited by the Council on Social Work Education. Currently there is no specific accreditation of psychiatric (or mental health) social work programs, although such a provision existed until 1960, when the Council on Social Work Education eliminated the accreditation of specialty curriculums (Ferguson, 1969).

The Professional Association

The organization representing social workers today is the National Association of Social Workers, formed in 1955, after three years of planning (Stroup, 1960). This body was antedated by both the American Association of Psychiatric Social Workers, established in 1926, and the Psychiatric Social Workers Club, affiliated with the American Association of Hospital Social Workers when the club became the Section on Psychiatric Social Work in 1922 (French, 1940). Membership in the National Association of Social Workers is available in several categories, including graduates of accredited master's degree and baccalaureate programs and social work students.

Major Mental Health Settings

Social workers are significantly involved in the professional staffing of each of the major mental health facility categories discussed in the following subsections. Some of the typical social worker functions are presented relative to these practice settings.

Veterans Administration

The Veterans Administration as a single entity employs the largest number of trained social workers in the United States. Social work staff are appointed to positions in general medical and surgical hospitals, neuropsychiatric hospitals, outpatient clinics, day hospitals, day treatment centers, and regional offices.

Social work staff in neuropsychiatric hospitals engage in a variety of professional functions and activities. These include conducting preadmission social service evaluations. This assessment by the social worker usually involves not only an interview with the veteran but also an interview with the person accompanying the veteran to the hospital. Often this is a family member—spouse, parent, or child. This psychosocial evaluation defines the problem for which hospitalization is being sought and assesses the family unit's functioning, particularly emphasizing supports that are available to the veteran. A competent preadmission evaluation by the social worker may result in the veteran's referral to another community resource such as a family service agency or mental health center. On the other hand, if hospitalization appears to be indicated—the social worker may admit the veteran directly but only a physician may deny admission—then the accompanying relative is helped to view the hospitalization and the potential outcome in a realistic way. The social worker draws an initial impression about the receptivity of the family for having the veteran back home. Thus, this preadmission evaluation is useful to the veteran, the relatives, and the staff in arriving at realistic expectations for hospital treatment.

In conformity with standards set forth by the Joint Commission on Accreditation of Hospitals, a treatment plan is worked out for the veteran, who signs the plan at admission or at a treatment planning conference. This requirement by the Veterans Administration safeguards the veteran's rights while facilitating a collaborative approach between the patient and the hospital staff.

Among the many professionals involved in mental health services, such as accountants and personnel specialists, social workers deal directly with patients or clients rather than support or facilitate direct services. The social worker in a Veterans Administration neuropsychiatric hospital may counsel patients individually or in groups and develop discharge plans with the veteran and family. Social workers often are responsible for making alternate community placements, matching individual veterans and their needs with community resources. Supervision and follow-up of the veteran's placement in the community setting may also be part of the social worker's responsibility.

Social workers assigned to regional office staffs typically are involved in providing a variety of services to veterans living in extramural environments, including their home and facilities like group and family care homes. These veterans include those who have been discharged from neuropsychiatric hospitals.

In a sense, the Veterans Administration clinical social worker is an aftercare agent, attentive to the veteran's problems and needs in the areas of income maintenance, housing, employment, and medical care. Understanding the community and its resources is basic to the social worker's role performance.

There are many other specialized activities in which a Veterans Administration social worker may be involved: staff supervision; administration of the social work service; needs assessment; and the development of needed community resources for the veteran. Social workers may carry primary responsibility for operating day treatment centers for veterans in urban areas.

While these social worker functions within the Veterans Administration are representative, they are far from being inclusive; furthermore, they are not exclusive functions in the Veterans Administration, as subsequent discussion will reveal.

Community Mental Health Centers

Social workers in community mental health centers are involved in virtually all the activity categories of the service elements. They engage in a variety of clinical and nonclinical tasks.

Clinical activities center around direct patient services such as inpatient care, outpatient care, emergency care, and partial hospitalization services. Some of the responsibilities include conducting intake interviews, providing individual counseling to clients, providing marital counseling, and providing family and other group counseling (see Chapter 5). Social workers may supervise or staff hot-line crisis services. Often, social workers are the numerically dominant profession in outpatient services—the element considered by many to be the backbone of any comprehensive, integrated array of mental health services.

Social workers also may serve as administrators or directors of community mental health centers or their various components (see Chapter 6). In the capacity of director, the social worker usually is responsible to a community board. Managing a complex organization entails hiring and firing staff; preparing the agency's budget; complying with federal, state, and local laws and policies; and a host of other activities. In studying the priorities and perspectives of administrators of mental health facilities (Callicutt, 1972), I discovered that the development of fiscal resources, including grants, was the major activity. Social work was the prevalent discipline among the administrators included in this study, although psychiatry, psychology, and hospital administration were also represented.

Increased attention is being given by community mental health centers to serving the chronically mentally ill. This shift is consistent with recommendations made by the President's Commission on Mental Health (1978). Community support arrangements along the lines conceived by Fairweather, Sanders, Cressler, and Maynard (1969) frequently put social workers in key roles in the planning, development, and operation of "Fairweather Lodges." Personnel work with a selected group of chronic mental patients in a hospital setting, prepare them to operate an income-producing business or service (janitorial services are typically chosen), and move them as a group into the community. This community arrangement is known as a Fairweather Lodge. A variety of extramural community supports are arranged: housing, transportation, health, and mental health services. In this role, the social worker is engaged in an array of planning and community organization activities, as well as in some supportive counseling.

Social workers often play prominent roles in the provision of services to other special or target populations, including alcohol and other drug abusers, the elderly, children, and minority groups. Among the helping professions, no single discipline has exclusive responsibility for specific problem areas or concerns. However, the Mental Health Systems Act of 1980 required that a member of the professional staff supervise the mental health care of every patient of a center. Here the key words are "professional staff," which includes social work personnel.

Emphasizing the importance of prevention, the Mental Retardation Facilities and Community Mental Health Centers Construction Act of 1963 and Amendments included consultation and education among the essential service elements of federally funded community mental health centers. The other four essential elements of service were inpatient, outpatient, partial hospitalization, and twenty-four-hour emergency services—all direct, clinical services. Consultation and education programs typically serve non-mental health professionals, including ministers and school teachers; these programs may take the form of in-service education for teachers or seminars for ministers.

Social workers are heavily involved in the consultation and education, training, and evaluation service elements. They may supervise or staff such programs. Consultation activities may be case centered or focused on a specific problem of other service providers, professionals, or agencies including the courts, probation and parole officers, the schools, and other health and social welfare personnel.

From the preceding discussion, it is clear that in the community mental health arena social workers hold a variety of professional positions in both clinical and nonclinical areas.

Outpatient Clinics

Child guidance clinics and other mental health clinics employ approximately one-fourth of the social workers practicing in mental health settings (National Institute of Mental Health, 1980). Social workers frequently conduct intake evaluations and counsel clients. They are knowledgeable about community resources and services and make referrals to other agencies. They may also hold administrative and supervisory positions. Because these clinics are outpatient service operations, they entail social work roles and responsibilities similar to those in other outpatient settings, such as in community mental health centers.

As a member of the classical mental health team—psychiatrist, psychologist, and social worker—the social worker participates in staffing conferences, which include the formulation of treatment programs for the client.

State and County Mental Hospitals

State and county mental hospitals have undergone significant changes since 1955, when the resident population in these facilities began to decline—a decline that has continued to the present. While the resident population began diminishing in 1955, the annual number of admissions to state mental hospitals increased yearly until 1971. Since then, admissions have decreased steadily each year.

Legal actions and court decisions have had a profound effect on these institutions. In some states, hospitals have been closed and community care mandated by the courts. The role of the courts in making social policy in many areas, including the mental health arena, is undeniable. Thus, state and county mental hospitals have had no choice but to respond to court decisions and orders. A community care approach, long a part of social work's orientation and philosophy, is increasingly their answer to court or-dered service requirements.

Social workers in state and county mental hospital settings perform many of the functions listed in the discussion of Veterans Administration facili-ties. They may be responsible for directing or staffing specialized units, including those for alcoholics, drug abusers, geriatric patients, and adoles-cents. In addition, state hospitals that offer outreach services often look to the social worker to provide both leadership and client services in this com-munity environment, which requires the utilization of community organi-zation and other social work skills.

Residential Treatment Centers

Administrative, supervisory, and clinical positions are filled by social work-ers in residential treatment centers for the emotionally disturbed. Social workers participate in admission evaluations and in staff conferences for planning treatment and discharge. They also provide counseling to clients individually and in groups. Counseling families and arranging follow-up services for discharged residents are other important functions.

Other Settings

Private mental hospitals, freestanding day/night facilities, and other mul-tiservice facilities combined account for about 7 percent of the full-time equivalent social work positions in mental health practice settings (National Institute of Mental Health, 1980). Social worker duties vary according to the individual settings. All these settings, however, use the social worker's expertise in family dynamics and community resources. (The emphasis on the client in the total environment characterizes the orientation of com-munity mental health, community medicine, holistic medicine, and tradi-tional social work practice.)

Future Trends

The Community Mental Health Centers Act of 1963 and Amendments have had a major impact on the development of mental health services in every state (see Chapter 2). The establishment of mental health centers in com-munities has created the need for personnel to staff them. Social workers are among the professionals most heavily utilized, as noted earlier in this chapter. Their training in direct practice (work with individuals, families, and small groups), community organization, administration, planning, and research uniquely qualifies them for this and alternate mental health settings (see Bevilacqua, 1980, and Morris, 1980).

Some states, with Massachusetts a prime example, are investing increased fiscal resources in the community mental health system, allowing for reductions in the state hospital population (Okin, 1979). Social workers should be in the forefront of these efforts, which are consonant with traditional social work values and require the social worker's expertise. The trend toward community mental health centers is likely to bring new attention to the field of social work and to encourage interdisciplinary research and methods.

While other professions share areas of expertise with social work, social work will continue to be a major contributor in areas in which it pioneered, including aftercare, preadmission screening, family casework, and community organization, including the development of self-help and mutual aid groups. Effective community service requires knowledge of the local population. Innovative training programs that combine course work and field instruction focused on specific groups such as the elderly are already in operation. This trend is likely to expand in the future.

In conclusion, as Mechanic (1980) pointed out, recent developments in mental health care in areas other than drug treatment have come from nonmedical disciplines. He credited social work with a long history of employing crisis intervention techniques. Underscoring the communtiy care thrust that has been frequently mentioned in this chapter, Mechanic noted that this practical management of patients "has been a traditional concern among social work agencies" (p. 181). In view of this record, it is reasonable to expect social workers to play a vital role in the future both in the wide array of traditional mental health settings and in alternate care programs for mental health clients.

REFERENCES

BEVILACQUA, J. J. "Social Work Dimensions in Mental Health Services." In J. W. Callicutt (ed.), *Health Care Issues in the 80's: Social Work's Contribution in Physical and Mental Health.* Arlington, Tex.: Graduate School of Social Work, University of Texas at Arlington, 1980.

CALLICUTT, J. W. "Maine Mental Health Agencies' Executives' Perspectives regarding Selected Problems, Prospects, and Programs." Research report submitted to the Maine Bureau of Mental Health, 1972.

CANNON, I. M. *Social Work in Hospitals* (new and rev. ed.). New York: Russell Sage, 1923.

DEUTSCH, A. *The Mentally Ill in America* (2d ed., rev. and enl.). New York: Columbia University Press, 1949.

FAIRWEATHER, G. W., SANDERS, D. H., CRESSLER, D. L., and MAYNARD, H. *Community Life for the Mentally Ill: An Alternative to Institutional Care.* Chicago: Aldine, 1969.

FERGUSON, E. A. *Social Work* (2d ed.). Philadelphia: Lippincott, 1969.

FRENCH, L. M. *Psychiatric Social Work.* New York: Commonwealth Fund, 1940.

GOLDSMITH, J. M. "Mental Health Services for Children." In J. B. Turner (ed.), *Encyclopedia of Social Work* (17th Issue), vol. 2. Washington, D.C.: National Association of Social Workers, 1977.

LEE, P. R., and KENWORTHY, M. E. *Mental Hygiene and Social Work.* New York: Commonwealth Fund, 1930.

MECHANIC, D. *Mental Health and Social Policy* (2d ed.). Englewood Cliffs: Prentice-Hall, 1980.

Mental Health Systems Act, P.L. 96–398, October 7, 1980.

Mental Retardation Facilities and Community Mental Health Centers Construction Act of 1963 and Amendments, P.L. 88–164, P.L. 89–105, P.L. 90–31, P.L. 90–574.

MORRIS, R. "Alternate Social Worker Roles in Health Care." In J. W. Callicutt (ed.), *Health Care Issues in the 80's: Social Work's Contribution in Physical and Mental Health.* Arlington, Tex.: Graduate School of Social Work, University of Texas at Arlington, 1980.

NACMAN, M. "Mental Health Services: Social Workers In." In J. B. Turner (ed.), *Encyclopedia of Social Work* (17th Issue), vol. 2. Washington, D.C.: National Association of Social Workers, 1977.

National Association of Social Workers. "Report of the Mental Health Task Force." National Association of Social Workers, 1979. Mimeographed.

National Institute of Mental Health. *Staffing of Mental Health Facilities, United States, 1976.* DHEW pub. no. (ADM) 78–522. Washington, D.C.: U.S. Government Printing Office, 1978.

———. Unpublished data, Division of Biometry and Epidemiology, National Institute of Mental Health, 1980.

OKIN, R. Address in *Proceedings, Governor's Conference on Mental Health.* Raleigh N.C.: Office of the Governor, 1979, pp 46–49.

ROONEY, W. S. "Military Social Services." In H. L. Lurie (ed.), *Encyclopedia of Social Work.* New York: National Association of Social Workers, 1965.

RUBIN, A. *Community Mental Health in the Social Work Curriculum.* New York: Council on Social Work Education, 1979.

———. *Statistics on Social Work Education in the United States: 1981.* New York: Council on Social Work Education, 1982.

SOUTHARD, E. E., and JARRETT, M. C. *The Kingdom of Evils.* New York: Macmillan, 1922.

STEVENSON, G. S. *Child Guidance Clinics.* New York: Commonwealth Fund, 1934.

STROUP, H. H. *Social Work: An Introduction to the Field.* New York: American, 1960.

WOODWARD, L. E. (ed.). *Psychiatric Social Workers and Mental Health.* New York: National Association of Social Workers, 1960.

PART TWO

Direct Services

The chapters contained in this section reflect a dominant system of curriculum organization in social work education. They also are representative of social work practice, revealing the variety of ways in which clinical functions are organized formally and shaped by theoretical and professional orientations. The decision to devote separate chapters to services to individuals and services to families and groups was based on a convention in the mental health field. However, we recognize that these approaches are complementary, not mutually exclusive.

Each chapter reviews historical highlights. In addition, Chapter 4 discusses the therapeutic techniques, theoretical orientations, social work roles, and mental health settings related to contemporary social work services to individuals. Ted R. Watkins also looks at nontraditional services, current trends, and future directions in this area. Chapter 5 explores the contributions of social work to family and group treatment. The authors' relational approach to family and group therapy, developed by Donald R. Bardill and elaborated by Benjamin E. Saunders for use in rural mental health settings, is a major focus of the chapter.

These authors speak from their extensive practice experience, as well as from their academic perspectives. Together they contribute not only to a more adequate understanding of contemporary direct practice services in the mental health arena but also to the knowledge base of the fields of social work and mental health.

CHAPTER 4

Services to Individuals

Ted R. Watkins

GESTALT PSYCHOLOGY and, more recently, systems theory speak to the interrelationships, indeed, the inseparability, of parts within a whole and of parts to the whole. This concept of mutuality and interdependence has been applied to mechanical, biological, ecological, and human interactional systems. It is equally relevant to thought systems or concepts. Any concept is related to, and defined by, the use of other concepts. The terms "mental health," "social work," and "services to individuals" appear deceptively simple but, in fact, each is a complex concept or thought system that is difficult, if not impossible, to separate from many other concepts or thought systems. How does one separate mental health from mental illness, emotional maturity, or social functioning? When does social casework directed toward enhancing social functioning become mental health work? How does one separate out services to individuals from the larger network of factors that contribute to the well-being of the individual, such as social change efforts, administration of services, or supervision and consultation?

Such complexities dictated certain limits on the scope of this chapter. For example, I give scant attention to child welfare services, family counseling, and medical social work, all of which have obvious mental health goals but are not generally classified as mental health resources. Similarly, a number of specialized mental health services for specific population groups have been omitted for the sake of brevity (e.g., counseling for homosexuals, women, the recently divorced or widowed, and stepfamilies). I also omitted the highly variable factor of educational prerequisites for social work in mental health settings. The reader may assume that the term "social worker" refers to an individual who has completed professional training specifically in social work at either the bachelor's, the master's, or the doctoral level. The phrase "services to individuals" denotes those activities whose target unit of intervention is the individual rather than the family, a larger social group, or society as a whole. The reference section at the end of the chapter reflects the major corroborating sources for the content, and the interested reader may turn to this list for more comprehensive coverage.

Social Work Applications in Mental Health

Social work is a relatively new profession, having emerged in the early 1900s out of Western civilization's long history of private and, more recently, public charitable activities. Initially serving as a link between needy individuals and groups and the material resources of the society, the field soon began to augment the dispensing of material resources with various efforts to assist the needy by offering advice, emotional support, and encouragement. While some social workers became social change agents through advocacy for the disadvantaged, others focused on casework—one-to-one services to individuals in need. Mary Richmond's *Social Diagnosis,* published in 1917, was the first compendium of the casework process. Using input from caseworkers representing several cities and diverse fields, Richmond explicated a tentative but concrete and comprehensive process of assessment of social functioning. She addressed the many dimensions of social interaction that contribute to adequate or inadequate social functioning, the caseworker's state of mind as a factor in assessment, the importance of context in understanding behavior, the impact of family and other social roles on mental well-being, and essentials of the interviewing process, including objectivity, empathy, utilization of the individual's strengths, and the interaction of personality and social environment. She concluded that the aims and process of casework are essentially the same regardless of the symptomatology of the client, though therapeutic procedures might necessarily differ. This first guide to social casework practice reflected the territory that social work was pioneering—the interaction between the individual and society.

The knowledge base of social work was developed both by borrowing from fields such as psychology, sociology, economics, medicine, law, and political science and by learning from social work practice. Social work has remained a profession of *application* of knowledge from diverse fields, rather than a discipline of theory and research only. The focus is still on the interaction of individuals and larger social systems.

Social work has long recognized that the individual in need is more than a victim of social problems. He is both an actor and a reactor. Casework has striven to enhance the social functioning of the individual through helping him use himself more effectively to find greater fulfillment of his needs for growth, self-esteem, and comfort within the context of his social reality. The individual's social adjustment and mental health are inseparable. Constructive social adjustment is both a cause and a result of mental health. Emotional disturbances that require mental health services are most often recognized when they manifest themselves in problematic interactions with others, such as excessive displays of hostility, possessiveness, guilt, or isolation. Even self-destructive behavior is related to unsatisfactory interpersonal relationships, such as a feeling of rejection by others, a sense of alienation from others, or a desire to punish another. Social casework specifically addresses the relationship between the individual and the other—whether family, friends, employers, and other individuals or social institutions such as schools, hospitals, and human services systems. Improvements in patterns of interaction with the social environment enhance the self-concept and mental health of the individual, while improvements in overall mental health result in better social functioning.

Of the mental health professions (traditionally identified as psychiatry, psychology, social work, and psychiatric nursing), social work has been the major advocate for the recognition and utilization of interpersonal relationships in the provision of mental health services (Torgerson, 1962). This focus on the individual in interaction with his social context remains central to social work and, to whatever extent there is differentiation among the mental health professions, distinguishes the social worker.

While there is a considerable amount of shared knowledge, skills, and perceptions among the mental health professions, along with much variation among the practitioners of each profession, social work is generally distinguished by its focus on the social dimension of the psychosocial field, as opposed to the intrapsychic, or psychological, dimension; by its emphasis on the healthy part of the individual, as opposed to pathology (thus the term "client" is generally used by social workers rather than the label "patient"); and by its efforts to change functioning rather than personality structure. Having neither the psychiatrist's tool of chemotherapy through which to bring about changes in the thought processes, feelings, and functioning of the client, nor the clinical psychologist's repertoire of psychological testing by which to see into the client's psyche, the social worker relies most heavily on his perceptions, judgments, and interactional skills in mental health treatment services.

Few research studies have compared the effectiveness of psychotherapy by profession, but available findings suggest that social work is at least as effective as the other mental health professions. Meltzoff and Kornreich (1970) noted that "there is no satisfactory evidence to indicate that one professional discipline is any more or less effective than the other" (p. 266). Sullivan, Miller, and Smelser (1958) compared outcomes in psychotherapy done by psychiatrists, psychologists, and social workers and found no significant differences. Frank (1979) stated, "The results of outcome research strongly suggest that more of the determinants of therapeutic success lie in the personal qualities of the patient and the therapist and in their interaction than in the therapeutic method" (p. 311). Strupp (1973), however, found professional differences among social work, psychology, and psychiatry in their interactional processes in response to a hypothetical case. Social workers gave significantly more responses that were reassuring, encouraging, and compassionate. Social work responses were also more accepting, understanding, and permissive and less directing; included less opinion and analysis; provided more clarification and reflection; expressed less passive rejection, disbelief, and ignoring of the client's request or complaint; and showed less antagonism, aggression, sarcasm, irony, and cynicism. Logically these findings would be expected if one accepts that (1) emotional and/or behavioral problems have their roots in earlier unsatisfying relationships or interactional patterns with the social environment; (2) the client's immediate life situation reflects past deficits or learning in that current social relationships are troublesome; and (3) the distinguishing characteristic of social work treatment is its offering of corrective and growth producing interpersonal experiences. Thus, social work services are immediately relevant to the factors underlying the client's emotional distress.

Within the social work framework of treatment of individuals with mental health problems via a social interactional intervention (i.e., assessing and treating the client in relation to his interactions with family, employers, or broader social systems), two differing philosophies of treatment have evolved; each has several variations and subspecialties.

The older of the two, the psychodynamic model, grew out of the vast contributions of Freudian psychoanalysis and ego psychology. The infusion of psychoanalytic theory into social work education and practice began in the 1920s; this perspective is still dominant, though far less accepted now than in earlier decades. Basic assumptions of the psychodynamic model are that (1) the individual has a unique personality structure that includes conflicting forces and that is relatively stable over time; (2) there are myriad unconscious elements in the personality that influence the individual's behavior; (3) relationships and experiences with significant others during early developmental years color one's perceptions of and shape one's responses to current interpersonal relationships; and (4) current and future social functioning can be improved through gaining insight into the causes and effects of one's distorted perceptions and inappropriate responses to current life experiences. Among the many variations that have emerged from this basic personality theory are transactional analysis, with its more easily understood terminology and its strictly social interactional focus; functionalism, based on Otto Rank's variations on the basic themes of Freud; and Gestalt therapy, emphasizing the inseparability of the physiological, psychological, and social dimensions of the individual.

The second major philosophy of social work treatment of individuals having mental health problems is behaviorism. Behaviorism, or social learning theory, attends to the observables in social interaction. Therefore, unconscious motivations, personality structure, insights, early life experiences, and feelings, being unobservable and unverifiable, are given little attention. Instead, the focus of behavioral therapy rests on specific actions of the client and the factors in the client's social environment that precede, accompany, and follow these behaviors. Behaviorism grew out of the animal research of Pavlov and others who explored stimulus-response phenomena. Behaviorism as currently used in social work is based largely on the theories and research in operant conditioning of B. F. Skinner, Joseph Wolpe's concept and techniques of reciprocal inhibition, and the modeling theory of Albert Bandura. There are perhaps as many variations among behaviorists as there are among psychodynamicists. Thomas (1977) identified the following schools of behaviorism: operant, relying primarily on reinforcement of desired behaviors; respondent, using classical Pavlovian conditioning; personalistic, combining behavioral therapy with personality assessment and theory; cognitive-symbolic, emphasizing cognitive and symbolic mediation and vicarious conditioning; specialists, who apply only a single behavioral technique; and eclectic, who draw from several empirically supported frames of reference. The basic assumptions of behavioral theory are that (1) behaviors are the critical element in one's social adaptation; (2) behaviors are learned, can be unlearned, and can be replaced by more effective (prosocial) behaviors; and (3) increasing the prosocial behaviors of a client will result in his receiving more positive responses from his social environment, thereby further promoting adaptive social functioning. Among the many subspecialties within the behavioral model are emphases on controlling the triggering (antecedent) events, controlling the consequences of a behavior (providing either rewarding or aversive consequences), modeling prosocial behaviors and thus extending the client's repertoire, and teaching self-control techniques. Goals and outcomes are relatively concrete and easily measurable, facilitating research on this approach; the result has been a rapid proliferation of literature on behavioral therapy.

Few mental health social workers are neutral in their opinions of these two orientations. Behaviorism took root in social work as a result of disenchantment in some quarters with psychodynamic theory and its limitations. However, behaviorism was initially poorly received by most practitioners, and an inordinate amount of antagonism existed between the advocates of the two philosophies from the mid-1960s to the mid-1970s. There is now increasing recognition of the value in both approaches. The extreme polarization is diminishing, and advocates of each model are increasingly adopting elements of the other. Psychodynamicists are using behavioral techniques when their psychosocial assessment justifies this approach, and behaviorists are increasingly acknowledging the importance of such nonobservables as emotions. It is apparent that the ends sought by the two groups are often compatible and equally relevant to social work's goal of enhancing the social functioning (however this notion is defined) of the individual. Saleebey (1975) presented an excellent analysis of the philosophical differences between the two approaches and suggested ways in which they enhance each other.

The Role of the Social Worker in Mental Health Services to Individuals

Consistent with social work's emphasis on the individual and his social environment, the social worker in mental health settings focuses on the client's cognitive, emotional, and behavioral responses to events in his life, especially interpersonal relationships. For the therapy to be most effective, the social worker must provide for the client an experience within the therapeutic process that offers a more constructive model of interpersonal interaction, which includes more reality based intellectual perceptions, emotional reactions, and behavioral responses. Consequently, the key to effective social work services to individuals in mental health settings is the relationship between social worker and client. The social worker has responsibility for developing and shaping this relationship.

The nature of the helping relationship is that of a partnership between two experts joining forces in an effort to strengthen the client's ability to react in a responsible, constructive manner to his life experiences; i.e., in a manner that supports his development and well-being without being destructive to others. This may include work on clarifying and reinterpreting negative events of the past so as to diminish their impact on present life experiences. The goal is to improve functioning in the present, using experiences of the past only as means of facilitating adjustment and bringing about more objective perceptions of the present.

The expertise of the client as a member of the partnership is his unique knowledge of his current life situation, past factors that may be affecting his current functioning, his personal goals, and his strengths and weaknesses. The contribution of the social worker is his professional expertise in the areas of individual growth and development, his understanding of human relationships, his knowledge of the therapeutic process, and his professional skills and techniques. An egalitarian relationship between social worker and client is needed in order to maximize the benefit of each person's expertise.

The major tools of the social worker are his knowledge and skill and his own personality. Knowledge and skill can be developed through formal education. Self-understanding and the ability to use one's self as a powerful force in the therapeutic relationship with the client are more difficult to acquire. Increasing his self-knowledge must be a goal of the social worker throughout his career. The very personal nature of the problems of the mental health client requires a great deal of risk taking on the part of the client to reveal his most intimate problems to a stranger. It is essential for the social worker, then, to be trustworthy—a confidant who can facilitate self-revelations on the client's part, treat intimate material with respect and confidentiality, be empathetic, and understand the client's meanings. Clearly, the social worker must be in control of his own responses to the client and the client's problem. Since clients come in an infinite variety of forms, requiring an infinite variety of responses from the social worker, the social worker must be very flexible in his reactions to others. He must be able to communicate warmth or distance, authority or nondirectiveness, concreteness or abstractness, abruptness or subtlety, aggressiveness or passivity, depending on the needs of a particular client at a unique point in time. Truax and Carkuff (1967) defined the key therapeutic variables as genuineness, accurate empathy, and nonpossessive warmth. Understanding these concepts is one thing; constructively implementing them is another. As the client is influenced by his own personality and past learning, so is the social worker. Some of the factors that the social worker must understand about himself are his attitude toward differences between himself and others, his need to be in control versus his ability to let others choose their own direction and their own rate of progress, his value system and his willingness to allow others to have divergent value systems, and his gut level responses to persons of another ethnic background, socioeconomic level, physical type, sex, age, intellectual level, and lifestyle.

A number of means are available to help the social worker develop greater self-understanding. Introspective ability is essential to all of them. An understanding of one's own life situation and one's responses to it can increase empathy with others. Clinical supervision and consultation with peers can be a rich source of feedback about the social worker's use of his personality. Personal therapy can be an invaluable tool in self-understanding, as can participation in a broad range of experiential workshops, training sessions, and encounter groups. A keen perception of the client's responses and feedback to the social worker can be of utmost value. Understanding of self is the foundation upon which one learns to use one's self in a constructive way in the relationship with the client. Clearly, the social worker cannot be an effective change agent in the life of a client until he understands himself.

After gaining an understanding of his motivations and values, the social worker needs to analyze the way he presents himself to, and is perceived by, the client. A warm personality can be hidden behind a cold, impassive facial expression. Training in communication skills is important here. Videotaping is extremely helpful in identifying deficiencies in the area of communicating with clients (Ivey, 1971).

The third step in the process of providing mental health services to individuals is assessment of the client. Assessment begins when the first bit of information about the client is perceived and continues throughout the process of working with the client. The data base for an assessment includes the objective reality of the problem; i.e., what event or situation has precipitated the client's coming to the social worker. The presenting problem may range from hallucinations to marital conflict to job dissatisfaction to phobias. Second, what is the significance of this problem to the client? Does the client view the presenting problem as a sign that he is falling apart, that he is inadequate, that he has failed, or that things are hopeless? This subjective reality, how the client interprets his crisis, has a greater impact on him than the crisis itself. Third, what is the background of the problem? How did it begin and in what context? What prior events fit into the development of the problem? Fourth, how is the presenting problem affecting the client's functioning? Is there a ripple effect, whereby one problem is creating difficulties in other areas? Fifth, how has the client attempted to cope with the problem and what success has attended his efforts? How have the important people in the client's life responded to his attempts to cope?

In the process of gathering these data from the client, the social worker is simultaneously making assessments on two levels. First, he is assessing the problem, both in terms of its immediate nature and in terms of basic issues that may be underlying the problem. For example, while the presenting problem may be a parent's inability to control the behavior of a child, an underlying problem might be the parent's general passivity and inability to set limits on other people. The second level of assessment concerns the client. Data for this assessment come from the client's physical appearance, means of communication (both verbal and nonverbal), and responses to his problem, to others in the environment, and to the interaction with the social worker. Relying on the assessment of the client and his problem, the social worker can begin to draw together a treatment plan based on what resources exist within the client and his social environment, as well as within the agency and the community at large. Additionally, an assessment is made of what obstacles are likely to impede the client's progress. These obstacles may include limitations in the client, his social environment, the agency, and the community at large.

The helping process also involves the ongoing relationship between social worker and client, the follow-through by both members of the team, and the feedback through the continuing therapy process. Outcome goals must be clear, though they may not always be identical for social worker and client. Client and social worker will usually agree upon certain task goals; however, the worker may have process goals that may or may not be disclosed to the client. For example, in addition to helping the client learn to discipline a child more effectively, the worker may have a hidden agenda of enhancing the client's self-esteem, with the end result that the client can be more appropriately assertive in general.

It is essential that the social worker in a mental health setting be familiar with psychiatric nomenclature and have a good grasp of the treatment implications of various diagnostic categories. Even in the most nontraditional mental health settings, it is imperative that the social worker know the difference between neurotic and psychotic characteristics, be able to form quick diagnostic impressions of the client, and respond appropriately to the degree and direction of psychopathology in the client. For example, techniques used to help the neurotic client understand the defense mechanisms and motivations that underlie his problem behavior, with the goal of less defensive and more reality based responses on the part of the client, may be extremely detrimental to the psychotic client whose personality structure is too chaotic or fragile to tolerate insight and confrontation. Similarly, attempts to relieve the neurotic client of guilt might be highly inappropriate in working with a sociopathic character disorder whose underlying problem may involve insufficient development of guilt or remorse. Thus, the clinical social worker in mental health settings must understand the client's personality.

The social worker and client in a mental health setting will experience an ongoing shifting of balance between support and confrontation. Emotional support is necessary for the development of rapport with the client and is the major ingredient of warmth and empathy. It is a necessary first step in the development of the therapeutic relationship. Confrontation is the process of bringing to the client's awareness ideas, perceptions, or emotions of which he previously had little knowledge. Thus, the client becomes more aware of emotions that he is acting out and gains new information about himself, others, resources, etc. Techniques for confrontation range from those that are minimally threatening, such as parroting or paraphrasing what the client has said, thereby enabling him to see himself in a new light; to more aggressive means, such as relabeling in less positive terms behaviors to which the client has attributed a positive definition. Confrontation is a means of feeding back information to the client about himself and his situation. Confrontation is likely to stimulate defensiveness, perhaps hostility and antagonism, and fear and hurt on the part of the client. The social worker must constantly gauge the reaction of the client to confrontation.

Skillful alternation by the social worker of support and confrontation can produce a layered pattern in therapy. With initial support, the client begins to establish rapport and identification with the social worker. Some confrontation can then be added to help the client gain understanding. As the client becomes threatened enough by that confrontation to start pulling away in the relationship, a new layer of support can be added, followed judiciously by more confrontation. This process leads the client forward through alternating encouragement and support for his strengths while stimulating him to new movement by confrontation. Too much support can result in a false sense of mastery on the part of the client and a slowed growth process. On the other hand, excessive confrontation may alienate the client so that he withdraws from treatment or resists the efforts of the social worker to help him.

Support in the social work process serves to aid in the establishment of rapport and trust with the social worker, increase the client's self-esteem and self-acceptance, reward appropriate behavior and constructive coping actions, and break the tension of conflict when confrontation becomes too strong. On the other hand, confrontation serves to increase the client's awareness of the inappropriateness of certain of his coping mechanisms, demonstrate alternative responses, and stimulate him to new, constructive action. Confrontation must be used exclusively for the client's benefit rather than for the social worker's expression of hostility. It must be relevant to the client's problem; it must be meted out in doses that the client can tolerate; and it must be presented in a form that makes sense to the client.

Mental Health Agency Function and Supportive Structures

Social work mental health services to individuals are greatly influenced by the agency setting in which they are provided. Various factors will both change the degree of influence of social work and shape the direction of services from the social worker; for example, does the setting provide residential, round-the-clock care, or is it an outpatient facility; is the agency funded by government, the community, or private sources; is social work the primary profession providing services or is it secondary to another profession such as psychiatry, the ministry, education, or business management? While the social worker is accountable to his clients, he is also accountable to the agency and its funding bodies.

Over a decade ago, Piliavin (1968) developed a theoretical model for the private entrepreneurship of social work. He noted the restraints that agency settings impose on the social worker, making the point that agency based social workers, as employees of organizations dominated by conservative interests, are impeded by agency policies from fulfilling their primary obligation to clients. He proposed that agencies be dissolved and that social workers work autonomously by request from clients, billing the government for services rendered, as medicine is practiced under some socialized systems. Thus, the social worker's accountability to the client would be strengthened, agency bureaucracy would be eliminated, and professional manpower now being used in administration would be freed for direct service.

Among the many flaws apparent in this proposal is the lack of recognition of the facilitative and supportive aspects of agency structure for the social worker. A social worker's efficiency and quality of service may be enhanced by the supervision, peer support, cumulative expertise, and procedural guidelines offered by an agency. While the agency setting may be either supportive or inhibiting to the practice of the individual social worker, it is the responsibility of the social work clinician to maximize the benefits and minimize the liabilities of being attached to a specific mental health agency. The following section discusses major types of agencies in which mental health services to individuals are provided by social workers, the usual role of social work, and the strengths and weaknesses of each of these settings. Social work roles will be discussed within the broad categories of treatment, ancillary services, and prevention. Treatment refers to the social worker's being the major change agent in the provision of direct psychotherapeutic services to the client. Ancillary social work services are those in which the social worker provides supportive services, such as bringing about change in significant others in the client's life (parents, spouse, etc.) or working with the client in limited areas (taking social history, aftercare planning, budget counseling, etc.) while another professional takes major psychotherapeutic responsibility for the case. Preventive services are those in which the major objective is to stimulate and nourish healthy social functioning or otherwise to prevent or halt deterioration of social functioning.

Institutional Settings

The institutional setting that comes first to mind in considering mental health service delivery is the large government supported hospital. Many of these institutions arose in the mid-nineteenth century as a result of efforts by Dorothea Dix and other advocates of humane treatment for the mentally ill. Originally intended to give humane custodial care to the mentally ill, often in idyllic settings, these institutions also served the purpose of removing the mentally ill from the social setting in which they had been disruptive.

With the growth of practical understanding in psychiatry, particularly the use of medication in the 1950s and 1960s, these institutions progressed from being mere warehouses of the mentally ill to treatment centers—at least in theory. Recent judicial decisions have mandated that treatment services be available to all patients in mental institutions. Although the U.S. Supreme Court ruled in *O'Conner v. Donaldson* (1975) that there is no legal requirement that treatment be provided for involuntarily committed persons, a number of lower court decisions have maintained the opposite (Glass, 1977; Zusman and Bertsch, 1975). There is a wide range in the quality of care of the mentally ill in these institutions, though certain characteristics are common to the majority of them. These characteristics include heavy reliance on milieu therapy (a strategy to make the daily living situation of the clients therapeutic through planned activities, interactions, etc.); relatively little individual attention and a high degree of depersonalization, reflective of the high client to staff ratio and large institutional size; and use of a multidisciplinary staff, representing a broad variety of disciplines working under the aegis of the medical profession.

Often the level of training of staff is in inverse relationship to the amount of direct contact with clients. Social workers may carry key therapeutic roles in these institutions, or they may provide indirect services to individual clients through coordination of staff, serving as unit administrators, etc. The increasing use of behavior modification techniques with hospitalized clients gives additional status to social workers who can plan, implement, or supervise such treatment methods. Vast numbers of clients per social worker in the institution make extensive contact with any one client unlikely. The social worker, however, as part of the intake team, may serve an extremely important function in helping the client understand the reasons for his hospitalization, the changes that he is expected to make, and the opportunities and resources available within the institution for making those changes.

As treatment proceeds, if the client is allowed to visit his family it is likely to be the social worker who helps him to assess the positive and negative aspects of his experiences at home and to plan for greater success next time. As discharge from the institution becomes imminent, the social worker will assume a key role in discharge planning, including preparing both the client and the family for their reunion if the client is to live with the family again; making other living arrangements for the client, if necessary; and preparing him for that living situation, in part by putting the client in contact with the community resources that he will need, such as employment placement, follow-up care, educational and training opportunities, or financial benefits. If the hospital offers its own aftercare services, these are most likely to be provided by a social worker, who monitors the client's progress, gives crisis counseling when the client encounters problems outside the institution, draws on further community resources as needed, and in general eases the transition back into community life.

Disadvantages of a large institution for the social worker include the extremely high ratio of clients to social workers, an inordinate amount of paperwork, sometimes unwieldy bureaucratic restrictions, and often low status of social work in the institution, which is viewed as a predominantly medical facility. On the other hand, round-the-clock care gives the social worker much more complete knowledge of a client, offers the opportunity to make significant changes in the client's total environment, and gives the social worker access to a whole range of personnel and material resources to use on behalf of the client.

Large private psychiatric hospitals have many traits in common with state institutions; however, their funding base generally consists of direct charges to the client or his family and benefits from the client's hospitalization insurance. This private funding, offered at a higher rate per client than public funding, often results in a much lower client to staff ratio, clients of a higher socioeconomic level, and shorter term, more intensive care. Many of these institutions are extremely innovative, attracting highly qualified and creative staff from a number of disciplines. While still medically dominated, private psychiatric institutions tend to use social workers more as primary therapists with individuals and groups than is true in state institutions. Social workers are almost always used for family therapy in these hospitals, as well as for ancillary services. Follow-up care is likely to be provided by psychiatrists on a private basis. While the status of being associated with a private hospital offers some rewards, social work is generally viewed as a secondary profession in this setting, so the social worker's status within the hospital may be low. The social worker's intimate working relationships with experts in other fields, the frequent use of private hospitals for training in various professions, and the predominance of affluent clients, for whom generally accepted mental health treatment seems to be particularly appropriate, make these settings excellent learning environments and provide challenging opportunities for creative therapeutic services. The psychodynamic model of treatment still reigns supreme in most private psychiatric hospitals.

Another institutional setting deserving special comment is the residential treatment center for children and adolescents. Many of the larger of these institutions began as orphanages or homes for dependent children but were converted into residential treatment settings for emotionally disturbed or behaviorally disruptive children and youth. Clients in these settings come from a wide variety of socioeconomic backgrounds and family patterns. These institutions may serve several hundred residents, or they may be small group homes, the current trend being toward small group home settings. In institutions for more severely mentally ill children, the medical model is still predominant. A wide range of activities, including formal academic schooling, is generally provided on the premises. Institutions for less severely distrubed children and adolescents are more likely to use social workers as the primary treatment personnel.

As a general rule, each child in the institution is assigned to a social worker, to whom he can turn for therapy and support as needed. Much of this one-to-one service focuses on relieving the pressure of traumatic past experiences through catharsis and on helping the child to view and respond to current situations through a reality base rather than through perceptions colored by past experiences. Group treatment and, to a lesser extent, family therapy are also generally a part of the program at these institutions. The range of services offered by a social worker to individuals in child care institutions is great, including preadmission interviewing and assessment and the admission decision; orientation of the child to the institution; psychotherapy or supportive counseling to the child, along with liaison and possibly counseling services for the parents; maintenance of communication with referring agencies; determination of privileges or restrictions for a particular child; case management and coordination of services needed by a particular child; monitoring of progress; and discharge planning, which may mean preparing the child and his family for reunion or making other living arrangements for the child.

While the stress related to dealing constantly with very active children and adolescents is high, this disadvantage is counterbalanced by the rewards of being part of a system that offers positive developmental experiences, as well as treatment for emotional problems. Since placement of children in these institutions generally comes through social agencies such as child welfare departments or juvenile courts, social workers serve a natural liaison purpose and tend to have rather high status in the institution.

Institutional settings pose some unique problems for the social worker. One of the greatest of these is the increased intensity of relationships among staff members. Institutional staffs may be divided along professional-paraprofessional lines and/or by professional discipline, with medicine, nursing, psychology, education, recreation, clergy, and social work sometimes all represented, all working with the same clientele, and each operating in the context of its unique philosophy, goals, techniques, and interests. Accordingly, rivalry and shifting alliances among staff are common.

In the outpatient setting, the treatment of the client by the social worker is a private affair between the two individuals involved, whereas in the institution many other staff members and residents are affected by decisions made in a particular case. Treatment decisions often require follow-through by houseparents, attendants, recreation therapists, or other staff members. For example, if the social worker probes into especially painful areas of a client's life in a psychotherapeutic interview, the resultant behavioral upheaval is likely to require several hours of special attention from all other staff in contact with the client. This makes the institutional social worker accountable not only to the client, the funding source, and the administration but also to staff members called upon to implement his decisions and, to some extent, to other residents of the institution, who will evaluate the services they are receiving in light of the client's treatment program. If a client is given more off campus privileges in recognition of a need to assume greater personal responsibility, other clients may act out in response to perceived favoritism. This, in turn may cause resentment in other staffs, who see the social worker as having started the problem.

Another characteristic of social work in institutional settings is the unusual degree of authority that the social worker has over the client's life. The very fact of institutionalization implies the client's inability to care for himself and his need for structure. The social worker becomes a part of that structure and is the instrumental part of it if he is the primary case manager or therapist. Consequently, the social worker cannot be an all-giving person but must set limits and monitor the client's behavior (Watkins, 1979). In institutional settings, more than any other mental health setting, the social worker is viewed as part of the system.

Large institutions usually are bureaucratic, with lengthy chains of command, complex accountability procedures, and detailed, often contradictory, policy statements. While sometimes irritating, these features provide a structure necessary for coherent functioning. In the midst of complex interactions among clients, several levels of staff, and numerous professional conflicts, structure may be very facilitative. The social worker who is administratively accountable to a direct supervisor, the chief social worker, the clinical director, and the institutional administrator will find comfort in written guidelines and formalized procedures. Often in such bereaucratic settings there is a considerable amount of flexibility for pursuing one's own interests as long as basic bureaucratic demands are met. The large program's many facets provide a range of options for research, innovation, and specialization.

Outpatient Services

The vast majority of mental health services to individuals are provided in outpatient settings such as mental health clinics, child guidance centers, family counseling agencies, or private offices. In these settings, the social worker is likely to be the primary therapist, although he may consult with psychiatrists, psychologists, or other professionals about the client's needs. Most often, individual clients are seen each week in hour-long sessions, with the social worker providing a range of services, including psychotherapy, advocacy, linking the client with other resources within the community, and intervention on the client's behalf with family members, employers, or other persons with whom the client may be having difficulty. The client population in these settings includes those who are receiving aftercare services following psychiatric hospitalization, psychotics who are able to maintain community functioning through supportive outpatient therapy, persons dependent on alcohol or drugs, the whole spectrum of neurotic personalities, court referred legal offenders, children and youths with school adjustment or other behavioral problems, families in conflict, and the entire range of individuals who are experiencing difficulty coping with life crises.

While the social worker is a representative of the agency that employs him, in outpatient settings there generally is minimal involvement with other parts of the social service delivery system in the worker-client relationship. The cost-effectiveness of using social workers as primary therapists in outpatient clinics makes social work a predominant profession in these facilities, although supervision and direction may be provided by psychiatrists or, infrequently, psychologists. The autonomy of the social worker in outpatient settings is enjoyed by many social workers; however, there are disadvantages to this system, too. The social worker has little or no access to other professionals who know his clients and can help in making assessments or developing treatment plans. With the exception of infrequent home or school visits or other collateral contacts, the social worker's knowledge of a client is restricted to what he can gain from periodic in-office interviews. Moreover, he has no control over other aspects of the client's life, which makes it difficult to observe either discrepancies between the client's verbalizations and his actual behavior or shifts in affect or behavior. This handicap may be considerable in the case of a client whose defenses prevent his being open with the social worker or a client in treatment under coercion who is distorting information in order to minimize the impact of treatment. Fortunately, most outpatient clients are voluntary, whether the setting is a community mental health center, private practice, or a family counseling agency. Consequently, most clients are highly motivated to change.

In past years these settings tended to rely heavily on psychodynamic theory and worked predominantly with middle-class clients. The community mental health movement, however, has increased the number of low-income and culturally diverse groups receiving outpatient treatment. Insight therapy is not well received by some of these groups, so there is currently considerable pressure on social workers to develop or utilize more group specific models of treatment. Consequently, there is increasing use of action oriented methods, which bring more immediate, visible results, such as behavioral management techniques; similarly, the insight process may be accelerated through the substitution of transactional analysis and directive counseling for more traditional, nondirective psychotherapy. While traditionalists may abhor these "band-aid" methods, the non-middle-class clients of outpatient services tend to be unsophisticated about psychotherapy, have little respect for the mystique of psychodynamic theory, and expect immediate help with their current crises rather than long-range changes in overall functioning. Thus, a diverse clientele requires flexibility on the part of the therapist, since a typical caseload includes some individuals needing supportive follow-up care, some who demand quick results in a specific area, and some who are seeking long-term growth.

The outpatient based social worker, if not in private practice, usually participates in regular supervisory conferences with a more experienced social worker or other mental health professional. The supervisor is both the link to the administration and, more important, a resource person for the development of knowledge, skills, and understanding. This function is especially important because interaction with other staff may be minimal except for informal contacts.

Partial Hospitalization Services

Partial hospitalization services lie somewhere between institutional and out-patient settings in that the client is in treatment several hours a day but also pursues routine activities either at home or on the job. This category in-cludes therapeutic day care and intense activities centers for children and adolescents. Day hospital programs are one type of partial hospitalization: the client spends evenings at home with his family but for several hours during the day receives recreational, occupational, group, or individual treatment at the institution. Night hospitalization, on the other hand, en-ables the client to continue working or going to school during the daytime; evenings are spent in the treatment program.

These settings provide more structure than do outpatient clinics but are less restrictive than inpatient settings and have many of the advantages of both. Partial hospitalization gives the social worker the opportunity to ob-serve the client in a variety of interactions with other staff and clients, yet this service does not isolate the client from normal interactional systems such as family or co-workers. Partial hospitalization often gives the client sufficient relief from stress and provides enough therapeutic service that full-time hospitalization can be avoided. Thus, it is a less drastic way of treating the client for whom outpatient services are inadequate. Partial hos-pitalization is also used as a bridge between inpatient and outpatient care; thus, the person who is being discharged from a hospital setting can move into a partial hospitalization program for a time to ease the transition into a normal life situation.

The role of the social worker in partial hospitalization usually includes intake procedures such as taking the social history, orienting the client to the program, and setting treatment goals; ongoing individual, group, and family treatment; and discharge planning and implementation, along with follow-up services. Because of the tenuous adjustment of clientele, social workers who provide direct services in partial hospitalization will do sup-portive casework, teach concrete coping skills, and facilitate environmental change by working with members of the client's family.

Partial hospitalization services usually have multidisciplinary staffs, with great flexibility in the division of labor. Administrative functions (team leadership, case management, etc.) may be performed by a social worker, psychiatrist, nurse, psychologist, or other professional. The status of each professional on the team is determined largely by the dynamics of the team. Consequently, the individual social worker largely determines his impact on the program by his contributions to the team effort.

The partial hospitalization program is seldom an autonomous service, as hospitals and outpatient clinics are likely to be. Such programs usually are outgrowths of inpatient or outpatient facilities. Viewed as a link in the continuity of care approach, the partial hospitalization service is highly compatible with the social work profession's function of bridging the gaps between systems.

Nontraditional Services

There are a number of additional types of settings in which the social worker provides direct mental health services to individuals; for example, private industry, correctional institutions, rehabilitation services, public schools and institutions of higher education, large churches, and general hospitals. The major goal of each of these settings is something other than the provision of mental health services, and the mental health social worker is employed to facilitate achievement of the major goals of the setting. For example, progressive businesses and industries have discovered that emotional problems (including temporary life crises) are a major cause of productivity decline among employees. An in-house mental health service to counsel employees can both increase the efficiency of the company and benefit the work force. In some cases, employee unions introduce mental health services as an additional benefit for workers.

On-the-job mental health services have the advantage of treating the individual in his natural environment. The employee can either seek counseling himself or be referred by a supervisor or union representative. However, the advantages of immediate access to this service are somewhat offset by the fear of many employees that through a breach of confidentiality their personal problems will become known to superiors or co-workers. Thus, extreme precautions are needed on the part of the social worker to maintain confidentiality in all aspects of this work. There is obviously less pressure to reveal confidential information if the mental health services are provided under union, as opposed to management, auspices.

Clients served in these settings tend to be functioning fairly well, as demonstrated by their being employed, and to be highly motivated, since they view the service as necessary to keeping or progressing in their jobs. Services here generally follow the model of outpatient mental health clinics or family service agencies. Social work is usually the major profession represented, and clients are a fairly homogeneous group.

Military social work is another example of mental health services aimed at enhancing or restoring the individual's productivity on the job. Professional social workers were incorporated into the military mental health services during World War II, following many years' reliance on civilian consultants. At present, each of the military branches has its own system of using military and civilian social workers to provide mental health and other social services. Military social workers with master's degrees hold officer rank, while assistants at a technician level are noncommissioned. The range of activity is broad, including assignment to inpatient hospital units, mental hospital clinics, and disciplinary barracks; services to families; and alcohol and drug abuse services. Status and salary, opportunity for mobility and exposure to multidisciplinary mental health teams, and outstanding fringe benefits attract many social workers to military careers. Bureaucratic constraints and limited autonomy in such areas as choice of location are seen as disadvantages by some.

Settings such as prisons or juvenile correctional institutions generally provide therapeutic services to a small percentage of their inmates who have evident psychopathology, as documented by psychological or psychiatric evaluations. Unless the social worker has some potent administrative input, as well as a therapeutic function, the prognosis for effective treatment is rather poor because the client is required to participate in treatment; incarceration has a very destructive and nontherapeutic impact; and psychotherapy is likely to make little difference in the client's current situation. It might even be argued that normality is disadvantageous in the typical correctional setting. Whereas insight into past experiences or present interactional problems may have little value in this situation, behavioral methods directed toward helping the client learn new ways of dealing with current stress, along with coping skills that could enable the inmate to avoid precipitating punitive action from the institution's staff or other inmates, may be beneficial. If provision is made for voluntary use of mental health services by inmates, there is a much greater likelihood of accomplishing meaningful change. In addition to carrying out direct therapeutic services, the social worker in correctional settings may be very valuable in providing ancillary services such as helping the family make maximum adjustment to the inmate's incarceration and easing the transition of the client back into a more normal life situation as discharge becomes imminent. Perhaps the greatest contribution social work can make is through administrative input in humanizing the institutional structure. While mental health services are drastically needed in these settings, their effectiveness is contingent upon an environment that fosters positive change in the individual.

Mental health services provided by social workers in schools aim primarily to support the goals of the institution. Clients referred for these services tend to be academic underachievers or students with behavioral problems. After assessing the situation, the social worker may focus on the student's relationship with his family, school personnel, or peers. School social workers generally are employed by the school system and therefore are accountable to the school administration; however, some schools provide such services through contract with outside agencies such as a family service or mental health agency. In these cases, the social worker is minimally accountable to the school system and has greater freedom to be an advocate for the student in conflicts involving school personnel; at the same time, however, the social worker will have less influence within the system because of his position as an outsider.

Social work in schools, like industrial social work, gives the social worker the opportunity to deal with the client in the client's natural environment; this minimizes the artificiality of the service and permits the social worker to see firsthand the way in which the client interacts with his social environment. Moreover, intervention during a key developmental period in the life of the client enables the social worker to have a profound impact upon the future well-being of the client. On the other hand, the student client may feel coerced and consequently resist the social worker's services, so that an initial objective of the social worker may be to persuade the client that therapy is worthwhile.

In progressive and flexible school systems, the social worker has the resources of the total system to bring to bear on the client's needs. However, if the system is rigid, the social worker may be caught in a bind between the needs of the client and the resistance of the system to changing in order to meet the client's needs. As with institutional mental health services, the social worker's efforts in schools reverberate throughout the system, requiring extreme diplomacy in relation to other school staff. Some school personnel may be initially hostile to the social worker, whom they view as encroaching on their territory. Recent legislation, such as P.L. 94–142, which mandates the provision of social and mental health services for handicapped children, will result in far greater utilization of social workers in school settings, particularly in cases involving children with learning handicaps. The school social worker needs skills not only in working with the individual client but also in working effectively with a larger system.

In any setting in which social workers are used primarily to meet the major goals of the host setting, there is great opportunity for the social worker to have a meaningful impact through humanizing a larger traditional system. Supportive resources are generally plentiful and the social worker has access to follow-up information to help him evaluate the effectiveness of his services. On the other hand, the social worker may feel isolated, being surrounded by personnel who are working toward goals quite different from his own and who may have negative views of the services of the social worker. Since social work is not the major profession in these settings, the social worker may worry that any mistake or public relations faux pas on his part will endanger not only his own status but also the status of his profession. Through successful efforts, however, in relation to both the client and the larger system, the social worker can expand the territory and the credibility of his profession in directions in which social work has much to offer.

The past two decades have seen a proliferation of social workers in private practice. The majority of private practice social work services are one-to-one counseling and psychotherapy. The realities of the provision of private mental health services at this time usually dictate that the social worker in private practice have consultation or supervision from a psychiatrist or other medical personnel. These restrictions are enforced through state licensing requirements and third-party payment policies. Consequently, many social workers in private practice work directly with a psychiatrist, who may refer the client to the social worker only after having done a psychiatric evaluation and diagnosis himself. The psychiatrist then assumes liability for the treatment services subsequently provided by the social worker. The psychiatrist may sign insurance claim forms, take care of billing and collection of fees, and pay the social worker for his services. More typically, a less formal arrangement between psychiatrist and social worker exists: the psychiatrist does not see the client directly but through periodic supervisory or consultative conferences with the social worker becomes acquainted with each case, monitors progress, and assumes liability for treatment. The social worker is responsible for providing all direct services to the client and collecting fees, but the psychiatrist signs insurance claim forms. There is a growing trend toward removing state requirements for medical supervision of private social work mental health services. This would give far greater autonomy to the social work clinician but require the profession to monitor itself carefully. In private practice, more than in any other area of direct service provision by social workers, a master's degree in social work, the completion of extensive practice experience, and documentation of expertise through licensing, certification, or registration are required.

Current Trends and the Future of Services to Individuals

A number of recent trends will shape the development of services to individuals in the future. Increasing emphasis on cost accountability, the broadening of services to diverse population groups, and the increase in knowledge of therapeutic services all highlight the impracticality of continued reliance on one-to-one therapy as the major mode of treatment in mental health. Use of family and group therapy will increase, although there has been considerable resistance to movement away from one-to-one therapy. It seems likely that in the future only those social work clinicians employed in private practice or by private clinics and hospitals will be able to continue relying on individual therapy as the major treatment modality. In community supported and public agencies, work with individuals in mental health is likely to consist exclusively of short-term crisis intervention, initial assessment, and transitional services toward family or group therapy. While the mental health social worker must continue to be highly skilled in work with individuals, he will need to develop equal expertise in family and group therapy.

The trend toward community mental health services is very likely to escalate. Increasingly, mental health services will be offered on the job and in day care and public school settings. The current trend for churches to use clinical social workers on their counseling staffs will expand. This movement away from traditional, isolated clinical settings will make services more accessible to clients and help remove much of the stigma attached to mental health services.

As mentioned in previous sections of this chapter, there has been a dramatic shift in recent years from almost total reliance on insight therapy to use of behavioral methods. The integration of these approaches will proceed along with the expansion of services to lower income and minority groups and the development of effective treatments for new client populations.

Recent years have seen a proliferation of nontraditional therapies that are receiving much public attention. Hypnosis, once reserved for use by medical practitioners, is gaining popularity among social workers, especially for the treatment of tension and habitual behaviors such as smoking and overeating. Biofeedback is being used by some behavioral social workers in teaching relaxation techniques to clients with a variety of tension related symptoms, including alcohol and drug abuse, high blood pressure, and chronic headaches. Psychodrama, dance, and music are being used to facilitate the client's self-expression and self-understanding. While such new therapies are often rather narrow in their applicability and frequently overgeneralized and oversold, they will be selectively integrated into the mainstream of psychotherapy. Thus, the tools available to the social work therapist will become more varied. The integration of mental and physical well-being, stressed by Gestalt therapists, seems to be inevitable in the mental health field.

There has been, and probably will continue to be, some breakdown in the boundaries separating the mental health professions. Universities are developing innovative graduate programs in marriage and family counseling, community psychology, counseling psychology, and pastoral counseling. There is great overlap between these emerging groups and clinical social work. One implication of the development of these programs is that if social work is to maintain its status as a major mental health profession, it must either lengthen its clinical training programs or narrow their focus. The need for mental health professionals will continue to rise in our increasingly complex society, and social work must simultaneously solidify and expand its knowledge base to meet the growing need.

REFERENCES

BEVILACQUA, J. J., and DORNAUER, P. F. "Military Social Work." In J. B. Turner (ed.), *Encyclopedia of Social Work* (17th ed.), vol. 2. Washington, D.C.: National Association of Social Workers, 1977.

COMPTON, B., and GALAWAY, B. *Social Work Processes* (rev. ed.). Homewood, Ill.: Dorsey, 1979.

DEMOLL, L., and ANDRADE, S. (eds.). *Mental Health for the People of Texas.* Austin: Hogg Foundation for Mental Health, 1978.

FERGUSON, E. *Social Work: An Introduction.* Philadelphia: Lippincott, 1975.

FINK, A. *The Field of Social Work* (7th ed.). New York: Holt, Rinehart & Winston, 1978.

FISCHER, J. *Effective Casework Practice: An Eclectic Approach.* New York: McGraw-Hill, 1978.

FRANK, J. D. "The Present Status of Outcome Studies." *Journal of Consulting and Clinical Psychology* 1979, *47*(2):311.

GERMAIN, C., and GITTERMAN, A. *The Life Model of Social Work Practice.* New York: Columbia University Press, 1980.

GLASS, K. "Right to Treatment: O'Conner v. Donaldson." *Health and Social Work* 1977, *2*(1):26–40.

HOLLIS, F. *Casework: A Psychosocial Therapy.* New York: Random House, 1966.

IVEY, A. E. *Microcounseling: Innovations in Interviewing Training.* Springfield, Ill.: Thomas, 1971.

MELTZOFF, J., and KORNREICH, M. *Research in Psychotherapy.* New York: Atherton, 1970.

MORALES, A., and SHEAFOR, B. *Social Work: A Profession of Many Faces* (2d ed.). Boston: Allyn & Bacon, 1980.

PERLMAN, H. H. *Social Casework: A Problem-Solving Process.* Chicago: University of Chicago Press, 1957.

PILIAVIN, I. "Restructuring the Provision of Social Services." *Social Work* 1968, *13*(1):34–41.

PINCUS, A., and MINAHAN, A. *Social Work Practice: Model and Method.* Itasca, Ill.: Peacock, 1973.

REID, W., and EPSTEIN, L. *Task-centered Practice.* New York: Columbia University Press, 1977.

RICHMOND, M. E. *Social Diagnosis.* New York: Russell Sage, 1917.

ROGERS, C. R., GENDLIN, E. T., KIESLER, D. J., and TRUAX, C. B. *The Therapeutic Relationship and Its Impact: A Study of Psychotherapy with Schizophrenics.* Madison, Wis.: University of Wisconsin Press, 1967.

SALEEBEY, D. "A Proposal to Merge Humanist and Behaviorist Perspectives." *Social Casework* 1975, *56*(8):468–479.

SCHWARTZ, A., and GOLDIAMOND, I. *Social Casework: A Behavioral Approach.* New York: Columbia University Press, 1975.

SMALLEY, R. *Theory for Social Work Practice.* New York: Columbia University Press, 1967.

STREAN, H. S. *Clinical Social Work: Theory and Practice.* New York: Free Press, 1979. (a)

———. *Psychoanalytic Theory and Social Work Practice.* New York: Free Press, 1979. (b)

STRUPP, H. H. *Psychotherapy: Clinical Research and Theoretical Issues.* New York: Aronson, 1973.

SULLIVAN, P. L., MILLER, C., and SMELSER, W. "Factors in Length of Stay and Progress in Psychotherapy." *Journal of Consulting Psychology* 1958, *22*(1):1–9.

————. (ed.). *The Socio-behavioral Approach and Applications to Social Work.* New York: Council on Social Work Education, 1967.

THOMAS, E. J. "Social Casework and Group Work: The Behavioral Modification Approach." In J. B. Turner (ed.), *Encyclopedia of Social Work* (17th ed.), vol. 2. Washington, D.C.: National Association of Social Workers, 1977.

TORGERSON, F. "Differentiating and Defining Casework and Psychotherapy." *Social Work* 1962, *7*(2):39–45.

TRUAX, C. B., and CARKHUFF, R. R. *Toward Effective Counseling and Psychotherapy.* Chicago: Aldine, 1967.

WATKINS, T. R. "The Comprehensive Community Mental Health Center as a Field Placement for Graduate Social Work Students." *Community Mental Health Journal* 1975, *11*(1):27–32.

————. "Staff Conflicts over Use of Authority in Residential Settings." *Child Welfare* 1979, *58*(3):205–215.

ZUSMAN, J., and BERTSCH, E. F. (eds.). *The Future Role of the State Hospital.* Toronto: Lexington, 1975.

CHAPTER 5

Services to Families and Groups

Donald R. Bardill
Benjamin E. Saunders

SERVICE TO FAMILY and other groups traditionally has been and remains a vital area of both social work practice and the mental health field. While specific data is unavailable, it is safe to say that family and group treatment have become standard intervention procedures in most mental health settings. The plethora of articles, books, tapes, workshops, and training programs which have flooded the mental health community during the past decade is convincing evidence that family and group treatment strategies are being widely used. Further, while the research evidence is far from complete, it is clear that family and group treatment not only is being used, but is being used successfully by mental health professionals (Gurman and Kniskern, 1981).

Now more than ever it is important for social workers in mental health to be familiar with the history, development, and current use of family and group techniques. The diversity of clients seen in mental health settings is overwhelming. Poor, middle-class, white, black, no education, graduate degrees, married, cohabiting, severely disturbed, mildly distressed, and so on all are descriptions of some of the clients mental health workers see. The problems of these clients (for example alcoholism, depression, childhood behavior problems, and marital troubles) and the mandates of community mental health (such as prevention, treatment, and maintenance) are equally varied. Family and group treatment has emerged as an important and effective technology workers can utilize in this diversity of clients, problems, and mandates.

This chapter explores the historical and contemporary involvement of social work with family and group treatment. Social workers have been involved in every stage of the growth and development of family and group treatment, contributing to both its theoretical and its practical maturation.

The first section examines the social work heritage of working with families and other types of groups. The second section describes the growth of the "family therapy movement" from the mid-1950s until the present time. Section three details the current involvement of social work with families and groups. The final section describes the relational approach to family and group therapy.

Several comments about the following presentation are in order. The theoretical and methodological development of family treatment and group treatment has been historically intertwined. Many, if not most, of the theoretical concepts and practice techniques of both areas are applicable to familial as well as nonfamilial groups. Indeed, historically much group work was done with families as natural groups (Wilson, 1976). Although the emphasis of this chapter is on families and the development of family therapy as a treatment modality, the reader is asked to remember the applicability of family group concepts and techniques to nonfamilial groups. Second, this chapter will concentrate on broad treatment issues rather than on special categories of clients (such as single-parent families, abusive or alcoholic parents, or low-income families). Finally, the focus of this chapter is more on treatment than on maintenance or support.

The Social Work Heritage

Social workers have been involved with families and groups from the earliest days of the profession. As Siporin (1980) stated: "Marriage and family therapy are traditional and basic social work services. Social workers have provided these services as part of the core of social work practice since the beginning of the profession" (p. 11). Ackerman, Beatman, and Sherman (1961) concurred: "Historically, the family has been the major focus of social work concern" (p. 1).

Wilson (1976) described the development of social work's involvement with both familial and nonfamilial groups since the nineteenth century. The profession of social work has always taken a family and group orientation to practice. Some would dispute Siporin's (1980) claim that the early work of social workers was therapy in the narrowest sense, but the point is clear. From the beginnings of the profession, familial and nonfamilial groups have been a primary target for intervention on the part of social workers.

The nature of the profession in the early days probably explains this family and group orientation. The "friendly visiting" of the workers took them into clients' homes where there was close contact with families. Much of their concern was focused on family relationships and welfare. The settlement houses of the nineteenth century also influenced the profession's orientation.

Few clients came by themselves to settlement houses. Instead, they came in twos or threes or larger groups. Their motivation was based on curiosity, rumor from school or neighborhood, consciousness of perplexing problems, or a desire for friendly visiting. In the beginning, the helpers just responded to what they faced. They did not say to themselves, "Ah ha, here is the structure of a natural group!" (Wilson, 1976, p. 3)

Therefore, the family and group orientation of the social work pioneers grew not out of theorizing about the efficacy of the method but out of contact with client problems, populations, and structures. Conceptualization followed.

Many of the techniques of the early social workers, particularly the friendly visitor movement, sound strangely modern in their tone. Siporin (1980) described the directions given to friendly visitors in his excellent review of marriage and family therapy in social work. Visitors were instructed to see the parents at the same time if possible (conjoint sessions). The importance of the father in the life of the family was emphasized at a time when the mother was the symbol of family life. And parental functions and responsibilities were described and many times instruction in parenting was given (family life education).

The work of Mary Richmond holds many modern conceptualizations about family dynamics, as well as practice techniques. Most striking is Richmond's (1917) directive that the family be taken as a whole. This unitary view of the family is analogous to modern family systems theory. Richmond also recognized that the family is part of a larger system that influences its functioning. This farsighted view was given expression in Richmond's system of "charitable cooperation," an early form of family networking, according to Siporin (1980).

In discussing the internal dynamics of the family, Richmond observed that the social and emotional bonds among family members have a strong impact on individual behavior. Therefore, she cautioned against interviewing family members alone and separately. She thought that efforts at individual treatment would fail without cooperation from the family (Montalvo, n.d.).

Richmond (1917) also developed a notion of family cohesion. She saw families as being on a continuum from low to high cohesion. "Degenerate" families were at the low cohesion end and the "best type of united" family was at the high end. While Richmond did not enunciate a concept of enmeshment (Minuchin, 1974), that is, a situation in which families tightly bounded together inhibit individual functioning, her concept of cohesion has been incorporated into the most recent theories of family assessment (e.g., Olson, Sprenkle, and Russell, 1979). Again, a modern family therapy concept was being used by social workers at the turn of the century in much the same way and for similar purposes as it is today.

Montalvo (n.d.) listed nine contributions from Richmond's work that have strikingly similar parallels in modern theory about the family and groups.

1. Self-identity is derived partly from the interaction and identification of the differences of individuals in groups.
2. The treatment of the family group offers the opportunity to introduce new information into the family system and thereby increase the possibility of correcting misperceptions.
3. The treatment of one member cannot be considered out of the family context without jeopardizing the treatment.
4. Relationships may be one of the main causes of family disruption and the means of recovery may be found in treating them directly.
5. Family diagnosis should consider the family's potential functioning as revealed by evidence of earlier stability in coping with social and economic stress.
6. Family cohesion may be developed and used as a working concept in treatment and diagnosis.
7. The worker should view the family as a whole and fashion treatment accordingly.
8. The worker's treatment role includes listening, observing, focusing, and supporting strengths in the family group as they are revealed in the therapeutic process.
9. Neither treatment of the individual member nor treatment of the family group should be regarded as preferable.

Certainly, Richmond was not the only social worker to develop concepts concerning families and groups that are still in use today (Siporin, 1980). People in other professions also were elaborating concepts, theories, and techniques that have been reinvented by modern theorists and practitioners (e.g., Adler, 1931; Burgess, 1926). Some would say that an industrious and creative reader could take the work of any early social scientist or practitioner and show how it preceded modern theoretical developments. It is clear that early social work, while not family or group therapy in the strictest sense, was oriented toward these modalities and developed many valuable conceptual and practice tools.

The 1920s was a time of conceptual and theoretical development in psychotherapeutic treatment. It was also during this period that social work expanded its client population to include those outside the low-income population. World War I brought social workers into contact with the upper classes. Social work itself was developing as a profession, and the role of the psychiatric social worker began to unfold. The alliance with psychiatry had two effects on social work with families and groups. First, it brought social work into contact with psychoanalytic theory. Second, the individual orientation of psychoanalytic theory tended to inhibit social work's attention to family systems in treatment settings (Quaranta, 1979).

As social work became more aligned with psychiatry, the development of family and group treatment was slowed but not stopped. Siporin (1956) stated that though social work overidentified with psychoanalysis and psychiatry, "social casework found scope for its continued concern with families in distress" (p. 167).

In the 1930s the impact of other professions was felt. Family sociology began to develop conceptual tools to deal with the family as a unit (Burgess, 1926; Nimkoff, 1934; Waller, 1938). Anthropology also contributed to the family orientation (Malinowski, 1929; Mead, 1935). In short, the needed conceptual tools for family and group treatment were taking shape.

During this same period psychiatry started to emphasize interpersonal and social influences on human behavior. The work of Harry Stack Sullivan, Karen Horney, and others revolutionized traditional psychoanalytic practice.

In the 1930s, then, social work began seriously to develop family and group casework on a theoretical level, adapting many concepts from other fields and the early social work tradition. The 1940s brought new challenges. Family casework, marital counseling, and group work all became typical social work practices. During this period, the psychiatric social work model came into full use. In this team approach, a psychiatrist would treat the disturbed client, while a social worker was responsible for the functioning of the family. Sophisticated methods of dealing with both familial and nonfamilial groups were developed. The 1940s laid the groundwork for the emergence of family therapy as a coherent model in the 1950s.

Recent Historical Perspective

The development of family and group casework during the first part of the twentieth century has been largely ignored by modern practitioners and theorists of family and group treatment. In particular, histories of the family therapy movement seem to begin in the mid-1950s, as though family therapy arose in a vacuum.

Guerin (1976), Bowen (1975), Erickson and Hogan (1976), and Okun and Rappaport (1980) all wrote histories with this bias. Each of their accounts focused on the role of psychiatry, detailing the creative contributions of many of the psychiatric pioneers of family therapy, such as Murray Bowen, Nathan Ackerman, Theodore Lidz, and Don Jackson. Few of these histories, however, acknowledged the important contributions of the social workers who had been integrally involved in the development of family therapy. While Bowen (1975), in his review, specifically noted the contributions of psychiatric social workers during the 1930s to family therapy, he concluded: "Most of the evidence favors the thesis that the family movement developed within psychiatry, that it was an outgrowth of psychoanalytic theory, and it was a part of a sequence of events after World War II" (p. 286).

Psychiatrists such as Bowen and Ackerman were strong forces in the development of family therapy, but they did not work alone. The Bowen, Dysinger, Brody, and Basamania (1978) paper presented at the 1957 annual meeting of the American Orthopsychiatric Association is regarded by some as the national debut of family therapy. Betty Basamania, a social worker who collaborated with Bowen in early research on schizophrenic families, made important contributions to the development of family theory (Basamania, 1961; Bowen, Dysinger, and Basamania, 1978; Bowen, Dysinger, Brody, and Basamania, 1978). Similarly, during this time Ackerman worked closely with Frances Beatman and Sanford Sherman, both social workers (see, e.g., Ackerman, Beatman, and Sherman, 1961, 1967). Although only the lead author of these various collaborative publications is well remembered, largely because of academic convention, the fact remains that social workers were involved in the development of many ideas often attributed to head psychiatrists of a research group. The reader who wants a clear understanding of the evolution of family therapy would be well served by reading the work of the co-authors, as well as of the first authors.

By 1960 the theoretical development of modern family therapy was well under way, and the social work profession was active in this process. For example, in 1958 *Social Casework* (vol. 39, no. 2–3) published a special issue on family casework in the interest of the child. Articles dealt with family diagnosis, family treatment, research with families, and social stresses on the family. In 1959 the same journal (vol. 40, no. 7) devoted another issue to the family, addressing family dynamics, family diagnosis, the application of social science concepts to family diagnosis, and research in the family. Many social workers were involved with families in therapeutic settings, and they published extensively on their methods and perspectives.

After 1960, sophisticated discussions of family therapy became common. In 1964 Virginia Satir, a social worker, published what might be called the first integrated system of family therapy for the broad therapeutic community. *Conjoint Family Therapy* is a classic still widely used. Also during this period Donald Bardill began his work at Walter Reed Army Hospital with distressed families (see, e.g., Bardill, 1963; Bardill and Bevilacqua, 1964). *Family Group Casework* (Bardill and Ryan, 1964) outlined what might be termed a uniquely social work approach to family therapy. Other social workers contributed to the theoretical growth of family therapy during the 1960s. Frances Scherz (1962, 1964) explored family diagnosis and treatment. Ceila Mitchell (1960, 1961, 1965, 1967) worked on many aspects of theory and technique. Lynn Hoffman, originally associated with the

Ackerman group, became a theoretical force in her own right (1981). Thus, during and immediately after the official birth of family therapy, social workers were integrally involved in refining both the theory and the practice of family therapy.

The late 1960s and 1970s saw the expansion of family therapy. The systems orientation was being applied in a variety of settings and with many types of problems. The literature of this period is rich with the contributions of social workers. For example, social workers were involved in applying the family orientation to marital problems (Bardill, 1966; Goodwin and Mudd, 1966; Luthman and Moxom, 1962), divorce counseling (Brown, 1976), and heterogeneous client populations (Aponte, 1976). Creative techniques such as family sculpting and choreography were being developed (Papp, 1976; Papp, Silverstein, and Carter, 1973). Sex therapy also became an area of social work practice.

Of course, psychiatry and psychology contributed to the growth of family treatment during this period, and other fields entered the domain of family services. For instance, the American Association for Marriage and Family Therapy grew into a professional, credential granting organization with a stated goal of developing marriage and family therapy into a distinct profession (Williamson, 1979). The American Personnel and Guidance Association supports counselors from the field of education, many of whom work with families (Williamson, 1979). Other professionals working in this area now include home economists, the clergy (pastoral counselors), educators, sociologists, lawyers, and nurses. Thus, the family, once the recognized domain of social work (Siporin, 1980), is now an area of practice for numerous professions. While social work contributed much to this field during the 1960s and thereafter, it also lost its near monopoly (Saunders, 1980).

The theoretical growth of family therapy has been phenomenal. A detailed review is beyond the scope of this chapter. However, several ideas that social workers had a hand in developing are particularly noteworthy.

The Family as a System

As discussed earlier, viewing the family as a social system is not a new idea to social work. Although the conceptual tools of systems theory were not available for the use of theoreticians in the 1920s, many of the traditional ideas of family casework fit nicely into systems theory.

The Family Dynamic as the Cause of Dysfunction

In the 1950s, as we have noted, the conceptual tools became available to operationalize the early ideas of social work and to mine the experience of social workers with families. The concept of homeostasis, developed primarily by the Jackson group (which included Satir), was particularly relevant to the idea of a family etiology for individual dysfunction (Jackson, 1965). Dysfunctions were now seen not as aberrations but as functional outcomes of the family dynamic. In this perspective, treatment that did not involve the family made no sense.

The Family as the Client

This idea was indeed revolutionary. Even though social workers previously had dealt with whole families in family casework, the organizing reason was always the illness of the individual patient. While the family might have been seen as causing the client's problem, treatment was still concentrated on the individual patient. Viewing the family itself as the client changed not only the focus of treatment but also its goal: curing the individual gave way to changing the family dynamic.

The Family as a System within Systems

Social work traditionally had reasoned that forces outside the family impinge on its functioning and may be the major cause of dysfunction. This perspective was a unique contribution by social work to the family therapy movement. Social workers also were trained to identify and use the resources of the larger social system in order to effect change in the family. The conceptual tools of systems theory allowed social workers to place their well-developed practice skills into a theoretical framework. In this context, techniques such as family networking, which Richmond had foreshadowed, and community involvement in family therapy evolved.

The idea of the family as a system within other systems also brings up the issue of the most appropriate unit of treatment. During the 1960s and 1970s family therapy was applied to many dysfunctions. Some therapists insisted that family therapy was the treatment of choice in nearly every situation. Others operated on the principle of least intervention: what unit of treatment—individual, dyad, family, family network, community—offers the greatest degree of success with the least amount of interference? This principle is one of social work's main contributions to family therapy.

Focus on Process

Emphasis on the process of interaction came directly from systems thinking. Proponents of this approach suggested that the family dynamic is revealed through the processes family members use in their lives together, rather than through the subjects of their problems. The family therapist is more concerned with who talks to whom than with what is being said. Most of the major research groups in the 1960s and 1970s worked on this principle, although the Jackson group also was concerned to some extent with content.

Morphostasis and Morphogenesis

A major innovation in the late 1960s and early 1970s concerned the homeostatic properties of the family system. As we noted earlier, the concept of family homeostasis was a working principle during the first years of the family therapy movement. According to this concept, which grew out of systems theory and functionalist sociology, family processes move to stability; that is, the family will organize itself into a stable pattern until something occurs to disrupt the equilibrium.

Speer (1970) and Wertheim (1973, 1975) argued for the morphogenic quality of the family system—its capacity to change and adapt. In fact, the developmental cycle of families requires that they do just that on a regular basis. Healthy families were now seen as having some degree of morphostasis for stability in their organization, along with the capacity easily to adjust to new situations.

Current Involvement

Family and group social work is a complex area that is best described by reviewing domain issues, theoretical issues, training, practice, and family policy.

Domain Issues

Social work's loss of domain in the family therapy area during the past two decades and the increase in competition over the provision of services to families were briefly described. This issue is highly relevant for the future of social work with families. Social work needs to examine its historical involvement in, and expertise with, families and organize its practice responsibilities to families in a systematic manner.

Gordon and Schutz (1977) proposed that social work with families is a "natural specialization." People tend to organize their lives around, and divide their time among, certain institutions (the family, employment, school, medical care, the community, etc.). Areas of practice evolve naturally out of these categories, and social work with families is thus centered on a naturally occurring group. Siporin (1980) went further: "There is a substantial consensus on a conception of family and marriage therapy as a legitimate area of specialization in social work practice" (p. 15). He argued that marriage and family therapy should be a specialty within social work practice, with workers formally accredited.

In 1974, 25 percent of the members of the American Association for Marriage and Family Therapy were social workers (Humphrey, 1977). This statistic indicates both the involvement of social workers in marriage and family therapy and the lack of support their own profession gives these specialists. At the same time, this figure reminds us that competition over the provision of services to families is intense. At present, the profession of social work is structurally ill equipped to maintain its traditional role in the family domain. Siporin (1980) offered three suggestions:

> First, it is evident that much greater recognition must be given to the rich and long tradition within social work of the provision of family and marriage therapy as basic social services. Second, there is a need to recognize that training for marriage and family therapy has been a core element in professional social work education since its inception and continues to have a central place in social work undergraduate and graduate programs. This is obscured to some extent by the conception of social work method as casework, group work, community organization, and so on. Third, it is therefore indicated that social work educational programs clarify and certify that such instruction is given. (P. 20)

Siporin closed his argument thus:

> Family and marriage therapy is regarded by many social work practitioners and educators as a distinct area of specialization. There is a need for accreditation that has not been met by the social work profession. (P. 21)

For social work to meet the challenge to its traditional place in family services will require organizational and educational restructuring and recognition of the field's expertise and heritage. The urgency of this need for accreditation is suggested by the failure of most graduate social workers to meet the educational requirements effective January 1, 1984, for clinical membership in the National Association of Social Workers.

Theoretical Issues

Social work continues to be a major force in the development of family therapy theory. Social workers sit on the editorial boards of many of the leading journals concerned with family therapy: *Family Process,* the *Journal of Marital and Family Therapy,* the *American Journal of Family Therapy,* and the *American Journal of Orthopsychiatry.* A quick survey of the principal direct practice journals in social work—*Social Work* and *Social Casework*—reveals that family issues are a primary concern for social workers.

One theoretical and practice notion currently receiving a great deal of attention is the place of paradox and paradoxical techniques in family therapy. Many of the innovators in this area have been social workers (e.g., Hoffman, 1981; Papp, 1980).

Watzlawick, Beavin, and Jackson (1967) defined paradox as a "contradiction that follows correct deductions from consistent premises" (p. 188). Dell (1981) noted that classical paradoxes create this contradiction because they are self-reflexive, that is, they comment on themselves. He used the example of Epimenides of Crete stating that "all Cretans are liars." The context of this statement (Epimenides is a Cretan) and the content of the message ("All Cretans are liars") set up a circular contradiction. If the statement is true, then it is false.

Paradoxical interventions, interventions that create circular contradictions for therapeutic purposes, have been used primarily in the strategic school of family therapy for the purpose of either increasing or decreasing the frequency and severity of a problem behavior within a family (Haley, 1976; Madanes, 1981). Typically, a contradiction is created by setting the context of therapy against a therapeutic instruction. The context of therapy is change. The family has come to the therapist for help and expects that he or she will do something to change how the family functions and to eliminate the symptomatic behavior of the identified patient. A typical paradoxical intervention, however, would prescribe the dysfunctional systemic patterns of the family, including the symptom. The family would be directed by the therapist to continue to do what it always has done, while the symptom bearer would be instructed to continue the problem behavior or even to exaggerate it. In effect, the family is instructed to get worse, not better. Now, if the family obeys the directive, they are acting against the context and purpose of therapy (change and improvement). If they disobey the directive, they must change their dysfunctional behavior, but against the therapist's wishes.

Papp (1980) concluded that paradoxical interventions are especially appropriate with defiant families, who continually fail to cooperate with the therapist. Paradoxical interventions capitalize on the family's defiance by setting up a situation in which to defy the therapist the family must change dysfunctional systemic patterns and the problem behavior. In compliant families, those who tend faithfully to carry out the therapist's instructions, obeying the paradoxical directive demonstrates to family members their control over problematic patterns and the presenting symptom.

Paradoxical interventions can be classified as very powerful but unpredictable tools. Use of paradox is a delicate matter and should probably only be attempted be experienced therapists. However, as theoretical and empirical study about this powerful idea continues, it may well develop into a relatively predictable technique for use by every family therapist.

Team approaches to family therapy are also part of the theoretical frontier. While co-therapy has been in use for many years, the team approach utilizes several therapists, who may or may not be in the therapy room. Papp (1980) described the "Greek chorus technique," in which team members behind a one-way mirror observe another team member conduct a therapy session. After the session, a team consultation occurs and the family receives a prescription, usually paradoxical in nature, for that week. Again, social workers are in the forefront here.

Training

Social work education has always offered instruction in family and group treatment. Siporin (1980) detailed the continual involvement of the social work educational system in preparing family therapists. In a survey of seventy-six of the eighty graduate schools of social work in 1975-1976, Siporin (1980) found that 90 percent of the schools reported that instruction in marriage and family therapy was given in their basic methods courses. In addition, 68 percent of the schools offered elective courses in family therapy, 33 percent offered electives in marriage therapy, and 46 percent offered elective courses that combined the two areas. Clearly, then, social work as a profession is involved in training students in marriage and family therapy. But, further information is needed on other available training opportunities. For instance, do students receive clinical supervision in marriage and family therapy? How many students receive placements at which training in family therapy is provided? Equally important, how many faculty at social work schools list family therapy as a specialty area?

Although none of the eight accredited graduate programs in family therapy listed by the American Association for Marriage and Family Therapy (1980) is offered by a school of social work (most are in schools of home economics, education, or sociology), many social workers lead workshops in family therapy or supervise family therapists in training. Furthermore, a 1980 survey revealed that many approved supervisors in marriage and family counseling were also social workers (American Association for Marriage and Family Therapy, 1980).

Finally, social workers are involved in formal projects to improve family and group treatment. For example, at the Florida State University School of Social Work a team of faculty and practitioners is studying and working with families as a unit of research and treatment.

Practice

The practice settings for family therapy by social workers vary widely. Agencies, large and small, are utilizing family and group treatment approaches with many types of problems. Of course, community mental health centers and other outpatient facilities are natural settings for the family approach. Indeed, social workers in most direct service settings—medical facilities, child welfare organizations, and alcoholism and drug abuse programs—are utilizing a family approach.

Family approaches have been successful in traditional client services: marital therapy, family life education, sex therapy, therapy with children, and divorce counseling. In addition, new applications have been developed. Anorexia nervosa has been treated successfully with family therapy (Minuchin, Rosman, and Baker, 1978). Asthma (Liebman, Minuchin, and Baker, 1974) and diabetes (Minuchin, Baker, Rosman, Liebman, Milman, and Todd, 1975) also have been amenable to family therapy. It is reasonable to expect that other dysfunctions will be fruitfully treated with family approaches.

One area that seems promising is the use of family and group approaches with low-income and minority clients. To date little work has been done in this area (Aponte, 1976; Minuchin, Montalvo, Guerney, Rosman, and Schumer, 1967), but efforts in this direction are appropriate for social work practice.

Family Policy

The emerging area of family policy is not related directly to the treatment of families and groups but is an area of social work that probably will have a great impact on the delivery of services to families. Although Americans traditionally have thought that government should not interfere in the lives of families, any government policy is family policy to the degree that it directly or indirectly affects family life (Leik and Hill, 1979; Moroney, 1979). Proponents of family policy argue that making certain aspects of policy explicit and comprehensive will in the long run improve services to families.

Many of the experts in the area of family policy are social workers. A recent issue of the *Journal of Marriage and the Family* devoted to family policy included several articles by social workers (Newcomb, 1979; Zimmerman, 1979; Zimmerman, Mattessich, and Leik, 1979). In 1979 the major journal of the profession, *Social Work,* published a special issue on family policy. Finally, Kamerman and Kahn (1978) and Rice (1977), all social workers, recently explored this area in monographs.

To conclude, the traditional partnership between social work and families extends beyond direct services. The construction of policies for families is also a concern of the profession. The future of family policy is uncertain, but it is noteworthy that social workers have pioneered in this area.

The Relational Approach
to Family and Group Therapy

The relational approach to family and group treatment is concerned with relationships between people and between social systems. It examines the "interconnectedness among the life systems in which a human being participates" (Bardill, 1976, p. 15). One assumption of this approach is that human behavior is influenced and guided not only by individual personality characteristics but also by the impact of social systems. Interactional processes between people work to organize and shape human behavior. In a family or group system, these interactional processes may be used to change dysfunctional behavior.

Within this theoretical context the family or the group becomes the client, the target of intervention, rather than the individual. The characteristic interactional processes of the family or group are of primary concern (Bardill and Ryan, 1973). The goal of therapy is to alter the perspective and interaction of the family or group members.

The first task of therapy is to identify the most appropriate social unit for intervention. Different problems and circumstances call for different approaches. The relevant unit for intervention may initially be an individual, a family system or subsystem (e.g., the marital dyad), an interpersonal system such as a group, or the community system. The second task of therapy is to identify the systems processes that are maintaining the dysfunctional behavior. Such assessments are ongoing tasks. As therapy progresses, the relevant unit for intervention may change from the family, to an individual, to the marital subsystem, and then back to the full family system. Concomitantly, the interactional processes of the family will change during the course of treatment. Therefore, assessment and intervention are not two separate parts of therapy.

Indeed, the very act of assessing a system affects that system and therefore has treatment implications. Additionally, any intervention will give the therapist new information to use. Consequently, the assessment-intervention dichotomy is false. The procedures of the relational approach should be viewed as techniques of both assessment and intervention.

The following discussion reviews the major notions that undergird the relational approach to family work. These ideas supplement other conceptual and practice approaches.

Life Stances

The relational approach considers human beings in relationship to four life realities: self, other, context, and spiritual.

Self. The self is the subjective world. It includes the sensory and cognitive experiences of human existence. Each person must relate to his or her own concept of what he or she is. Critical to human functioning is the degree of participation of the self with the external world.

Other. The other is everything, organic and inorganic, that is not self. Of special concern are the other human beings who are a primary influence on the person's existence.

Context. Context is the perceived organization and structure of reality, or the way each person views the relationships between self and other. "Contextual factors such as values, beliefs, and expectations are learned and serve as a frame of reference for making meaning out of events" (Bardill, 1977, p. 10).

Spiritual. The spiritual reality serves as an organizing frame for self, other, and context. For example, the Christian concept of love is the basic life principle for some people.

The four life realities constitute an organizing structure for human perception and behavior. Recognizing the broad and controversial nature of spiritual reality, we focus in this brief presentation on self, other, and context.

People tend to establish a life stance, a patterned way of relating to others and to life in general. This complex but identifiable manner of living depends upon the relative emphasis placed on the life realities.

Generally, people who regularly account for the life realities of self, other, and context in their human transactions are likely to exhibit a range of appropriate behaviors and to live in a functional way. While there is no one who fully and completely occupies a single life stance at all times, troubled individuals are usually rigid and restricted in their stance toward life. Typically, these people diminish, ignore, or deny one or more of the life realities in their contacts with other people.

Figure 5.1 depicts three dysfunctional life stances. Figure 5.1b may be termed the submissing life stance. People who live in this manner typically diminish the self. Figure 5.1c is the aggressing life stance. This person discounts the reality of the other, showing little respect for fellow human beings. Figure 5.1d is the emoter life stance. Here contextual realities of life are ignored. The person typically overreacts to others, highlights subjective feelings, and ignores rules and regulations.

Use of life stance diagrams is valuable in two ways. First, the therapist is able to gain information about the functioning of each person within the

Figure 5.1.   Life Stances

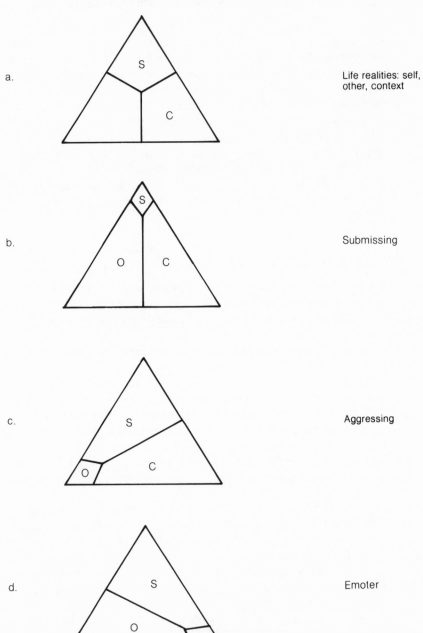

a.   Life realities: self, other, context

b.   Submissing

c.   Aggressing

d.   Emoter

relevant unit of treatment (e.g., the family system). The life stance approach helps the therapist organize the assessment of each individual. Second, by examining the relational connections among the life stances, i.e., how the life stances of family members match up, the therapist can begin to understand family relationships. For example, a person with an aggressing life stance will relate differently to a person with a submissing life stance and a person with an emoter life stance.

In a therapy session, family members may be asked to draw their own life stance or their perception of another family member's stance. There are two benefits to this procedure. First, family members are able to see how their various life stances fit together and begin better to understand their own family process. Second, the process of constructing life stances can reveal much to the therapist. For example, construction of life stance diagrams allows the therapist to view the organization of the family in action. Who leads the family? Whose ideas are discounted? Who speaks for other members? This process in itself is valuable in addition to yielding other information.

Genogram

The genogram, a concise representation of a family and its history, can be used by the therapist "to elucidate and organize facts and characteristics of the family, and dissect the emotional processes in a way that pinpoints the trouble spots in the relationship system" (Guerin and Pendagast, 1976, p. 450). The genogram serves to place the nuclear family within the context of its family history. The therapist is able to assimilate a great many facts about the family and explore possible relational patterns in the extended family system. Figure 5.2 illustrates a family genogram.

Like the life stance diagram, the family genogram has value both in providing concrete information and in revealing the family process. The therapist may seek to assess the characteristics of the extended family. Are its constituent families typically large or small, similar or different? Are there significant events such as deaths or divorces? How does the family go about providing this information to the therapist? Who is the family switchboard—the person who keeps track of birthdays and other important dates?

Life Space Diagrams

Life space diagrams represent family members' perceptions of family relationships. Each family member is asked to draw a representation of the relationships in the family; rectangles indicate family members. The size

Figure 5.2.   The Family Genogram

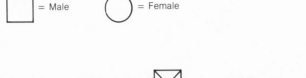

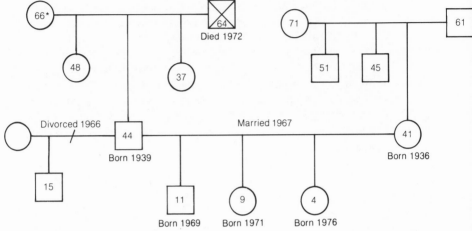

*Indicates age.

and placement of each rectangle is determined by the individual family member. The therapist may ask for diagrams depicting the family as it is, how it was in the past, or how each family member would like the family to be. The family members may then be asked to share their life space diagram with the rest of the family and the therapist. Figure 5.3 is a typical life space diagram.

Life space diagrams offer the therapist much information on family functioning. The differences and similarities in the perceptions of each member about the family dynamics serve to paint a picture of how the family operates. As is the case with life stances and genograms, the process of constructing and sharing life space diagrams is very important. Family members can begin to understand how they are viewed by other members of the family and can comment on these views. The therapist is able to observe how the family incorporates this information. Does the family as a whole diminish the importance of the information? Do members agree or disagree? Do they plan to take action on the basis of the new infor-

Figure 5.3.   Life Spaces

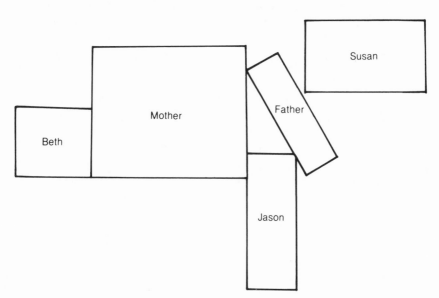

mation? The therapist can then utilize these insights in subsequent therapy sessions.

Family life space diagrams are similar in purpose to family sculpting and choreography (Papp, 1976; Papp et al., 1973; Simon, 1972). However, life space diagrams do not require the physical space that sculpting or choreography demands (a prime concern in many agency settings). Also, for many families life space diagrams are not as emotionally threatening as sculpting since they involve representations rather than the clients themselves. (This is not to diminish the usefulness of either sculpting or choreography. Indeed, the relational approach uses both these techniques, which are powerful tools for revealing the process of family interaction. But for a rigid family system, sculpting or choreography may be too threatening. Life space diagrams accomplish much the same purpose and most families readily participate.)

The Family Grid

A family system displays patterned behavior in much the same fashion that an individual does. Life stance analysis, the genogram, and life space diagrams help the therapist understand the patterned behaviors of a client family. Assimilating this material into a coherent picture of family functioning is a primary therapeutic task. The family grid serves this purpose.

Three primary dimensions of the grid identify family functioning: boundary, organization, and feedback. A family system displays a psychological boundary that identifies who and what is and is not regarded as family. The nature of this boundary may be viewed along a continuum from solid to amorphous, with two relevant intermediate points, permeable and open. Families whose boundary tends toward the solid end of the continuum have a strong we-they attitude. They may even seek to isolate themselves from people who are not in the family. Families with more amorphous boundaries may have no sense of cohesion. Each individual is on his or her own and family life is not very important.

A family also displays a sense of organization, the implicit and explicit rules about behavior by which family members operate. The family may be loosely or rigidly organized. Two relevant intermediate points on this continuum are structured and flexible. The rigidly organized family operates in an atmosphere of control. Family behavior is prescribed and there are definite expectations for every family member in almost every situation. Rules are precisely set and enforced. These rigid rules may be covert or overt but are nevertheless potent. This type of family is not open to change. The loosely organized family has very few, if any, rules. There are no real family roles and behavior is individually directed and uncoordinated. Family life is unpredictable and somewhat chaotic.

Finally, the family system relies on an organized and predictable pattern of feedback about the state of the family at any given time. Feedback may be viewed as either communications designed to keep the system in a stable, unchanging pattern or communications designed to shift or change the pattern. To be functional, a family must have both stability producing and change producing feedback.

The two dimensions of boundary and organization may be placed on horizontal and vertical axes to form a grid (see Figure 5.4). The grid is divided into four quadrants: A, B, C, and D. Each quadrant has characteristics determined by the two basic dimensions. The relational approach takes the position that fixity at any extreme on the family grid is dysfunctional. A loosely organized family is as dysfunctional as a rigidly organized one. Thus, the most dysfunctional families would be in the corners of the grid (shaded in Figure 5.4). Families that fall toward the center of the grid, the zone of functionality, may exhibit some of the extreme qualities of their quadrant but they are better able to adapt to new situations.

Family feedback becomes very important during assessment and intervention. Utilizing the information gained during therapy sessions, the therapist can place the client family on the family grid. This makes the goals of therapy much clearer, and the therapist can then use appropriate techniques to move the dysfunctional family toward the center. For example, a family with a solid boundary and a rigid organization needs to be brought into closer contact with the community and to loosen its rules. In this case,

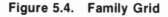

Figure 5.4. Family Grid

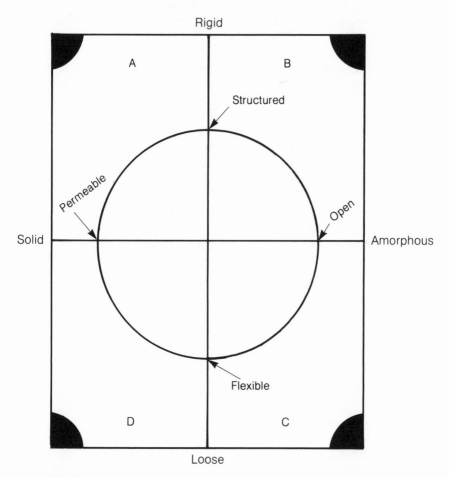

the therapist might seek to get individual family members involved with extrafamilial groups.

Conclusion

Work with families and groups is a traditional and basic area of social work practice. Social workers have been involved with familial and nonfamilial groups since the beginning of the profession. Many ideas advanced by the pioneers of social work foreshadowed the contributions of modern theorists.

During the past two decades social workers have refined and utilized family oriented approaches to therapy. For example, social workers have become involved in systems therapy with married couples, divorcing couples, and families. At the same time, other fields—home economics, education, sociology, and psychology—have challenged social work's preeminence in family services.

Nevertheless, social work continues to be involved with families. Some social workers have proposed that marriage and family therapy be recognized as a specialty within social work and that accreditation procedures be implemented. Social workers are active in the theoretical development of family treatment, in research and training, and in practice. In addition, social work is contributing to the new area of family policy.

The relational approach to family and group therapy focuses on the relationships between family or group members. Tools such as life stances, genograms, life space diagrams, and the family grid are used in both assessment and intervention. Techniques of therapy are derived from the understanding gained through these procedures.

Social work with families should play an even greater role in direct services in the future, as more types of problems are seen as amenable to treatment with a family or group approach.

REFERENCES

ACKERMAN, N. W., BEATMAN, F. L., and SHERMAN, S. N. (eds.). *Exploring the Base for Family Therapy.* New York: Family Service Association of America, 1961.

————— (eds.). *Expanding Theory and Practice in Family Therapy.* New York: Family Service Association of America, 1967.

ADLER, A. *What Life Should Mean to You.* New York: Putnam, 1931.

American Association for Marriage and Family Therapy. "AAMFT Accredited Graduate Programs." *Journal of Marital and Family Therapy* 1980, *6*(2):248–249.

—————. *1980 Register.* Upland, Calif.: American Association for Marriage and Family Therapy, 1980.

APONTE, H. J. "Underorganization in the Poor Family." In P. J. Guerin, Jr. (ed.), *Family Therapy.* New York: Gardner, 1976.

BARDILL, D. R. "Family Therapy in an Army Mental Hygiene Clinic." *Social Casework* 1963, *44*(8):452–457.

—————. "A Relationship-Focused Approach to Marital Problems." *Social Work* 1966, *11*(3):70–77.

—————. "The Making of a Person: A Psycho-social Analysis." *Social Thought* 1976 *6*(1):15–26.

—————. Relational Thinking and Person Abuse. *Social Work* 1977, *22*(0):10–12.

BARDILL, D. R., and BEVILACQUA, J. J. "Family Interviewing by Two Caseworkers." *Social Casework* 1964, *45*(5):278–282.

BARDILL, D. R., and RYAN, F. J. *Family Group Casework* (rev. ed.). Washington, D.C.: National Association of Social Workers, 1973.

BASAMANIA, B. "The Family as the Unit of Study and Treatment, Workshop, 1959; The Emotional Life of the Family: Inferences for Social Casework." *American Journal of Orthopsychiatry* 1961, *31*(1):74–86.

BOWEN, M. "Family Therapy after Twenty Years." In S. Arieti (ed.), *American Handbook of Psychiatry* (vol. 5). New York: Basic Books, 1975; reprinted in M. Bowen (ed.), *Family Therapy in Clinical Practice*. New York: Aronson, 1978.

BOWEN, M., DYSINGER, R. H., and BASAMANIA, B. "The Role of the Father in Families with a Schizophrenic Patient." *American Journal of Psychiatry* 1959, *115,* 1017–1020; reprinted in M. Bowen (ed.), *Family Therapy in Clinical Practice*. New York: Aronson, 1978.

BOWEN, M., DYSINGER, R. H., BRODY, W. M., and BASAMANIA, B. "Study and Treatment of Five Hospitalized Families Each with a Psychotic Member." Paper given at the annual meeting of the American Orthopsychiatric Association, Chicago, March 1957; reprinted in M. Bowen (ed.), *Family Therapy in Clinical Practice*. New York: Aronson, 1978.

BROWN, E. M. "Divorce Counseling." In D. H. L. Olson (ed.), *Treating Relationships*. Lake Mills, Iowa: Graphic, 1976.

BURGESS, E. F. "The Family as a Unity of Interacting Personalities." *The Family* 1926, *7*(7):3–9.

DELL, P. F. "Some Irreverent Thoughts on Paradox." *Family Process* 1981, *20*(1):37–42.

ERICKSON, G. D., and HOGAN, T. P. *Family Therapy: An Introduction to Theory and Technique*. New York: Aronson, 1976.

GOODWIN, H. M., and MUDD, E. M. "Marriage Counseling: Methods and Goals." *Comprehensive Psychiatry* 1966, *7*(5):450–462.

GORDON, W. E., and SHUTZ, M. L. "A Natural Basis for Social Work Specialization." *Social Work* 1977, *22*(5):422–427.

GUERIN, P. J., JR., "Family Therapy: The First Twenty-five years." In P. J. Guerin, Jr. (ed.), *Family Therapy*. New York: Gardner, 1976.

GUERIN, P. J., JR., and PENDAGAST, E. G. "Evaluation of Family System and Genogram." In P. J. Guerin, Jr. (ed.), *Family Therapy*. New York: Gardner, 1976.

GURMAN, A. S., and KNISKERN, D. P. (eds.). *Handbook of Family Therapy*. New York: Branner/Mazel, 1981.

HALEY, J. *Problem-Solving Therapy*. New York: Harper & Row, 1976.

HOFFMAN, L. *Foundations of Family Therapy*. New York: Basic Books, 1981.

HUMPHREY, F. "Family Services: Family Treatment." In J. B. Turner (ed.), *Encyclopedia of Social Work,* 17th Issue, vol. 1. Washington, D.C.: National Association of Social Workers, 1977.

JACKSON, D. D. "The Study of the Family." *Family Process* 1965, *4*(1):1–20.

KADUSHIN, A. "Social Work and the American Family Then and Now, 1920–1978." *Smith College Studies in Social Work* 1978, *49*(1):3–24.

KAMERMAN, S. B., and KAHN, A. J. *Family Policy: Government and Families in Fourteen Countries*. New York: Columbia University Press, 1978.

LEIK, R. K., and HILL, R. "What Price National Family Policy for Families?" *Journal of Marriage and the Family* 1979, *41*(5):457–459.

LIEBMAN, R., MINUCHIN, S., and BAKER, L. "The Use of Structural Family Therapy in the Treatment of Intractable Asthma." *American Journal of Psychiatry* 1974, *131*(6):535–540.

LUTHMAN, S. G., and MOXOM, J. "Diagnostic Classifications and Treatment Techniques in Marriage Counseling." *Family Process* 1962, *1*(2):253–264.

MADANES, C. *Strategic Family Therapy.* San Francisco: Jossey–Bass, 1981.

MALINOWSKI, B. *The Sexual Life of Savages in Northwestern Melanesia.* New York: Liveright, 1929.

MEAD, M. *Sex and Temperament in Three Primitive Societies.* New York: Dell, 1935.

MINUCHIN, S. *Families and Family Therapy.* Cambridge: Harvard University Press, 1974.

MINUCHIN, S., BAKER, L., ROSMAN, B. L., LIEBMAN, R., MILMAN, L., and TODD, T. C. "A Conceptual Model of Psychosomatic Illness in Children." *Archives of General Psychiatry* 1975, *32*(9):1031–1038.

MINUCHIN, S., MONTALVO, B. GUERNEY, B. G., ROSMAN, B. L., and SCHVMER, B. G. *Families of the Slums.* New York: Basic Books, 1967.

MINUCHIN, S., ROSMAN, B. L., and BAKER, L. *Psychosomatic Families.* Cambridge: Harvard University Press, 1978.

MITCHELL, C. B. "The Use of Family Sessions in Diagnosis and Treatment of Disturbance in Children." *Social Casework* 1960, *41*(6):283–290.

———. "A Casework Approach to Disturbed Families." In N. W. Ackerman, F. L. Beatman, and S. N. Sherman (eds.), *Exploring the Base for Family Therapy.* New York: Family Service Association of America, 1961.

———. "Integrative Therapy of the Family Unit." *Social Casework* 1965, *46*(2):63–69.

———. "Problems and Principles in Family Therapy." In N. W. Ackerman, F. L. Beatman, and S. N. Sherman (eds.), *Expanding Theory and Practice in Family Therapy.* New York: Family Service Association of America, 1967.

MONTALVO, F. "The Family as the the Context of Treatment." Manuscript, n.d. Worden School of Social Service, Our Lady of the Lake University, San Antonio.

MORONEY, R. M. "The Issue of Family Policy: Do We Know Enough to Take Action?" *Journal of Marriage and the Family* 1979, *41*(3):461–463.

NEWCOMB, P. R. "Cohabitation in America: An Assessment of Consequences." *Journal of Marriage and the Family* 1979, *41*(3):597–603.

NIMKOFF, M. F. *The Family.* Boston: Houghton Mifflin, 1934.

OKUN, B. F., and RAPPAPORT, L. J. *Working with Families.* North Scituate, Mass.: Duxbury, 1980.

OLSON, D. H., SPRENKLE, D. H., and RUSSELL, C. S. "Circumplex Model of Marital and Family Systems Part I: Cohesion and Adaptability Dimension, Family Types, and Clinical Applications." *Family Process* 1979, *18*(1):3–28.

PAPP, P. "Family Choreography." In P. J. Guerin, Jr. (ed.), *Family Therapy.* New York: Gardner, 1976.

———. "The Greek Chorus and Other Techniques of Family Therapy." *Family Process* 1980, *19*(1):45–58.

PAPP, P., SILVERSTEIN, O., and CARTER, E. "Family Sculpting in Preventative Work with 'Well Families.'" *Family Process* 1973, *12*(2):197–212.

Quaranta, M. A. "The Family as the Unit of Attention in Social Work." *Smith College Studies in Social Work* 1979, *6*(1):16–18.

Rice, R. M. *American Family Policy: Content and Context.* New York: Family Service Association of America, 1977.

Richmond, M. E. *Social Diagnosis.* New York: Russell Sage, 1917.

Saunders, B. E. "Social Work with Families: An Analysis of Domain Issues." Paper given at the annual meeting of the Southeastern Council on Family Relations, Mobile, Alabama, March 1980.

Scherz, F. H. "Multiple-Client Interviewing: Treatment Implications." *Social Casework* 1962, *43*(3):111–113.

———. "Exploring the Use of Family Interviews in Diagnosis." *Social Casework* 1964, *45*(4):209–215.

Simon, R. M. "Sculpting the Family." *Family Process* 1972, *11*(1):49–57.

Siporin, M. "Family-Centered Casework in a Psychiatric Setting." *Social Casework* 1956, *37*(4):167–174.

———. "Marriage and Family Therapy in Social Work." *Social Casework* 1980, *61*(1):11–21.

Speer, D. "Family Systems: Morphostasis and Morphogenesis, or 'Is Homeostasis Enough?'" *Family Process* 1970, *9*(3):259–278.

Waller, W. *The Family: A Dynamic Interpretation.* New York: Cordon, 1938.

Watzlawick, P., Beavin, J., and Jackson, D. D. *Pragmatics of Human Communication.* New York: Norton, 1967.

Wertheim, E. "Family Unit Therapy and the Science and Typology of Family Systems." *Family Process* 1973, *12*(4):361–376.

———. "The Science and Typology of Family Systems. Part II: Further Theoretical and Practical Considerations." *Family Process* 1975, *14*(3):285–308.

Williamson, D. S. "Board or Bored?" *American Association for Marriage and Family Therapy Newsletter* 1979, (September): 2–7.

Wilson, G. "From Practice to Theory: A Personalized History." In R. W. Roberts and H. Northern (eds.), *Theories of Social Work with Groups.* New York: Columbia University Press, 1976.

Zimmerman, S. L. "Policy, Social Policy, and Family Policy: Concepts, Concerns, and Analytical Tools." *Journal of Marriage and the Family* 1979, *41*(6):487–496.

Zimmerman, S. L., Mattessich, P., and Leik, R. "Legislators' Attitudes towards Family Policy." *Journal of Marriage and the Family* 1979, *41*(6):507–518.

PART THREE

Community Practice

The organization of this section is based on the rationale that community practice methods fall into the categories of administration, planning, and community organization. Although these areas often overlap, we decided to approach them separately in order best to exploit the knowledge and skills of experts in the three areas.

Thomas J. Kane's chapter on administration addresses the major roles and substantive issues in the field today. He discusses such diverse tasks as board selection and education and termination of staff. Trends and issues discussed include marketing, performance contracting, and staff incentive programs.

Louis E. DeMoll taps his reservoir of experience as a teacher and mental health planner in identifying and discussing mental health planning activities and requirements in both governmental and nongovernmental contexts, including state mental health agencies, statewide citizens' organizations, and local community mental health agencies. He reviews a number of key issues, such as citizen participation in mental health planning.

Mark Tarail explores the development of community organization in social work and the rise of the community mental health movement. He also discusses selected principles and concepts of community organization in mental health; for example, task orientation versus process orientation, the integration of fact-finding with action, and community involvement. The chapter emphasizes neighborhood participation in service planning, program implementation, and political action to support local mental health facilities.

CHAPTER 6

Administration

Thomas J. Kane

THE SIGNIFICANCE of administration in the organization, development, and delivery of social services has been widely acknowledged during the past fifteen years. This recognition is reflected in the increased attention given to administration in graduate schools of social work.

> The keystone for optimum efficiency and effectiveness in the achievement of social work goals in a changing society is the administration of social work programs. . . . the quality and nature of their administration determine in large measure both the potential for and the realization of their success. (Schatz, 1970, p. 1)

Social work administration draws on behavioral, political, social science, and economic knowledge, as well as on business and public administration methods. There is considerable disagreement, however, as to whether social work administration is merely the application of administrative techniques in a social work setting or is, in fact, a specific social work method.

Schwartz (1970) suggested that the social work administrator is a change agent managing a change system. He likened the social work executive to the social caseworker and supervisor, but the administrator relates indirectly to the agency's clients through the agency's social work system by

> influencing the determination of agency objectives and policy, marshalling resources, combining them in ways designed to aid the client system, coordinating staff to the end of offering a unified and appropriate approach to the client system, evaluating, and influencing the improvement of performance standards. (P. 26)

Schwartz also noted the convergence between social work administration and community organization.

In fact, social work administrators in mental health traditionally emerge from the ranks of practitioners, bringing with them greater clinical than management skills. According to Kendall, despite efforts to develop administrative training programs at the master's and doctoral levels, as well as institutes and workshops for practitioners, "none of this has been enough and all of it has come too late in the educational experience to provide enough administrators for middle as well as top management positions in the social welfare field" (quoted in Schatz, 1970, p. 111). The following review of social work administration in mental health must be read against this background.

Mental Health Administration

In the past, mental health administration was whatever the superintendent of a state hospital said that it was (Yolles, 1975). The shift to accountability and professional management in mental health settings has been accompanied and promoted by the shift from institutional to community services. (Chapter 2 explores the evolution of comprehensive, community based mental health systems). The trend toward deinstitutionalization presents the mental health administrator with a dramatic set of creative challenges. He now faces the task of developing new systems of care that provide diversified treatment approaches; require community support services; depend on community acceptance of deviant behavior; emphasize prevention and early intervention; and expand the client population from acutely mentally ill adults to families and children disturbed by emotional problems and social stresses.

The shift from a medically dominated and institutionally based service delivery system to a community based system of care has opened up administrative positions in mental health, long filled by psychiatry, to the other helping professions—social work and psychology in particular (Beigel, 1975). In 1976 only 30 percent of center directors were psychiatrists; 21 percent, psychologists; 31 percent, social workers; and 18 percent, other professionals.

While the shift to community services has complicated the role of the mental health administrator, it has not been accompanied by an increase in his administrative knowledge and competence: administrators "are often promoted to executive positions by virtue of their seniority or clinical abilities and are attracted to administration by salary, status or the power to get things done" (Feldman, 1973, p. xi). In community based mental health organizations, then, the chief executive officer is customarily a senior clinician, with more administrative experience than training, whose professional identity as a caseworker may be incompatible with effective management. Feldman (1978) noted that

> for the mental health professional who is also an administrator [the clinician's caring, supportive role is] often inconsistent with the exercise of power—the directive and perhaps authoritative stance sometimes necessary for successful administration. (P. 142)

Levinson and Klerman (1972) further suggested that the reluctance to use organizational power may lead mental health administrators to overemphasize collective decisionmaking and to tackle problems through process rather than action.

On the other hand, the clinician brings to the administration of mental health services sensitivity, understanding of group dynamics, and firsthand experience in the very services that he is to administer. Indeed, the shift from institutional to community based services encourages the application of social work values, perspectives, and skills to mental health administration. Mental health administration must take into account the agency's product—clinical services; the consumer—an emotionally troubled or mentally ill client; the service provider—mental health professionals, including social workers, psychologists, and medical personnel; and the funding source, either government or private organization. Thus, the clinician, properly grounded in administrative skills and thoroughly acquainted with the resources, objectives, and values of the agency, maybe uniquely qualified to administer a mental health services facility.

Feldman (1978b) challenged this view. He would prefer "undisciplined" mental health professionals, with a degree in mental health rather than the traditional disciplines of psychiatry, psychology, social work, etc. He also advocated separate professional training for the mental health administrator. Yolles (1975) supported this position, arguing that not enough attention is being paid to this "new breed."

Others, however, call for the management of mental health services by professional managers (Burgess, 1974). This position has gained considerable support among those who think that mental health professionals are "caught up in a circular, self reinforcing system of interlocking needs, a system that has bound us into relatively fixed and self serving patterns of behavior" (Feldman, 1978b, p. 91). Proponents of professional management argue that the clinical value system of an administrator prejudices his judgment and renders him unable objectively to administer the resources entrusted to him.

This view merits attention. The history of human services contains numerous examples of conflicts both among professionals and among programs: psychiatrists versus psychologists, clinicians versus consultants, inpatient versus outpatient services, prevention versus rehabilitation, etc.

A systems orientation, characteristic of professional managers, can help the administrator understand the interaction of program and staff components.

The clinical administrator, in dealing with other staff, must carefully distinguish between therapeutic and management skills. The available research indicates that effective management by clinical administrators requires, not empathy, but the same skills that industrial managers use: definition of job expectations, performance feedback, goal setting, and resource allocation (Steger, 1973; Wagner, 1975).

Klerman and Levinson (1972) further stressed the vulnerability of the clinical administrator in dealing with the external environment. The clinician is taught that human service organizations operate on a cooperative model and that their primary goal is to provide services. Studies reveal (Kane, 1972) and experience suggests that the primary motivation in interorganizational activity is power. The reluctance of clinicians to wield power may compromise their effectiveness in this critical area of administration. An essential component in a systems approach to service delivery is the organization's ability to negotiate advantageous interorganizational transactions.

In sum, the success of the clinical administrator model requires the synthesis of clinical and management values, skills, and techniques. The clinical administrator must understand that his clinical perspective—enhancing the social functioning and quality of life of the organization's clients—can best be supported by the development and implementation of sound organizational principles and processes. This requires a significant transition for the direct service provider and support from the profession in the form of training opportunities and explicit endorsement of the administrator's management functions.

Operational Planning

Planning must be considered an integral part of the administrative process. It has been dangerously commonplace in the health and human services for planning and management functions to become separate and even antagonistic. The public accountability requirements of these fields has led to the establishment of oversight organizations such as health systems agencies, state health coordinating councils, and regional planning organizations, all of which are concerned more with regulation than with planning. The mushrooming of these organizations is largely a product of the failure of health and human service systems to take planning seriously. Administrators can safely assume that the more and better planning they do within their organizations, the less planning will be done for them, the more self-determination they will enjoy, and the more relevant will be their organizations' activities to organizational goals.

There are a number of theoretical approaches to mental health planning. Selection will depend upon the perspective and skills of the administrator and/or planner, as well as the characteristics of the environment in which the planning takes place. Littlestone (1973) described a number of planning theories:

1. rational planning—focuses on the demographic characteristics of the population and uses professional planning technology, process, and decisionmaking
2. community organization—mobilizes the community to plan for it-self, with planners serving as technical consultants
3. advocacy—mobilizes potential consumers of services to provide leadership in a planning process that tends to dictate action in response to the planning effort
4. social policy—planning from top to bottom begins with policy decisions dictating activities
5. systems analysis—focuses on the interconnecting components of the client and service system and attempts to address multiple dimensions simultaneously

The approach to planning depends heavily on the developmental stage of the organization. Diamond (1974) identified five basic steps in developing a community mental health center: (1) creating an organization, (2) designing a service delivery system, (3) obtaining community approval, (4) developing trusting relationships with funding sources, and (5) developing responsive programs. The process of initiating an organization will obviously call for greater emphasis on community organization and advocacy planning and afford social workers in mental health administration a unique opportunity to practice skills basic to their field. (In fact, however, one of the major deficiencies in mental health planning has been the absence of effective community organization and advocacy [Levine, 1970].)

Scobie (1971) underlined the primacy of citizen participation in planning. Community involvement is appropriate, in his view, in goal identification, resource analysis, development of a planning body, development of an action system, development of a supportive constituency, analysis of alternative courses of action, and creation of feedback mechanisms. Citizen participation is a thread that must weave through any effective planning process in mental health. Yet it is not at all uncommon for mental health administrators, social workers included, to see planning as an end in itself rather than a means to an end—delivery of needed, quality services to clients.

For the mental health administrator who must integrate operational planning into his basic administrative role, the focus will be both intraorganizational and interorganizational. A systems approach assists the administrator in assessing the likely impact that a decision in any one component of his organization will have on another component (Hutcheson, 1969). This is particularly important in organizations with programs that address special populations (children, the elderly, the chronically ill) and serve extensive catchment areas (e.g., rural communities). Any plan for emergency services, for example, will have a profound impact both on the utilization of inpatient services and on the stability of aftercare programs.

The social worker in mental health administration brings with him a special sensitivity to a systems approach to planning: social work traditionally has looked at the client in his environment. At the same time, the social worker in administration must learn to integrate planning and executive decisionmaking, which may be an unfamiliar responsibility.

Financial Management

Many trends have converged to curtail public funding of mental health services: growing national concern around the spiraling costs of health care in general, federal policy shifts, and abuses associated with deinstitutionalization in some areas. The overall impact of these trends, however, has been far more positive than negative. They have forced mental health administrators to manage rather than preside, and they have forced staff to become product, rather than process, oriented.

The mental health administrator today works in an economy of scarcity. He must recognize that there will never be enough resources to do the job that needs to be done. At the same time, the public will hold him accountable for efficient resource utilization. These constraints will influence everything he does as administrator.

The typical administrator is not competent to provide the sophisticated fiscal management needed in mental health agencies. He must hire a financial expert, who assumes day-to-day responsibility for fiscal management and provides the administrator with the information necessary to guide decisionmaking. However, ultimate fiscal accountability remains with the administrator.

Financial decisions affect not only the business aspects of the organization but also the delivery of care and the direction of the organization (Silver, 1974). The role of the administrator in a mental health agency is to integrate organizational, economic, and mental health factors. This job is complicated by federal money policies. Community mental health programs were expected, over time, to generate financial resources to replace the federal funds used to set them up and finance early programs. In fact, the withdrawal of federal support has resulted in cutbacks in nondirect (nonreimbursable) services such as consultation and education, cornerstones of the community mental health program. This usually has been followed by a retrenchment of certain direct services, a decrease in access to services through the closing of some facilities, a reduction of quality control and program evaluation activities, and an expansion of less costly group therapy (1980).

The financial management challenge in mental health administration today is to reverse this pattern by timely decisions that will prepare the organization to survive the loss of federal support. Several strategies are appropriate here.

Appropriate Staffing

In order to maximize income from third-party payors, it is critical to know which staff will be reimbursed for which services. For example, in most states, private insurance carriers, Medicare, and Medicaid will reimburse only those services provided by psychiatrists, Ph.D. psychologists, MSWs, and master's degree psychiatric nurses. On the other hand, a contract for all center services (Title XX, or eligible provider status for the center) guarantees reimbursal of any and all staff services.

Workable and Profitable Fee Schedule

The typical mental health program applies a sliding fee scale. In my experience, this approach encourages clients and staff to agree on minimal fees and results in insufficient client income (Kane, Meyer, and Andre, 1979). Staff social workers and other direct service providers generally are reluctant to discuss and collect fees for services. Therefore, the agency must routinely make a complete assessment of client resources and use a formula for fee setting that leaves little discretion to the clinician. The system must be so monitored that any substantial deviation from the standard fee structure requires administrative approval.

Client fees are critically important in an era of public funding cutbacks. Indeed, this revenue source may make the financial growth of the agency possible.

High Clinical Productivity

It is not uncommon in mental health centers, particularly those in the earlier stages of federal funding, for clinical staff to spend no more than one-third of their time in direct services. The irony is that in most instances, both administration and staff are oblivious to this fact while feeling overworked.

Given this situation, it will be virtually impossible to effect change without a reporting system that documents staff activity and provides a mechanism for monitoring clinical productivity. There is convincing evidence and experience suggests that given a mechanism for documenting and monitoring their performance, clinical staff can be made aware of their output and be assisted in reaching a mutually acceptable standard.

Program Budgeting

One of the features associated with federal grant support for community mental health centers is the failure of staff to feel or take responsibility for the financial health of the programs they serve. This deficiency has been reinforced by budgetary approaches that focus on total organizational performance. Separate program evaluation and budgeting would counteract this tendency and give the administrator the information needed to discriminate between financially successful and unsuccessful services and to stimulate productive problem-solving (Feldman, 1973).

Program planning budgeting (PPB) provides the decisionmaker with a systematic and comprehensive comparison of costs and benefits of alternative approaches to meeting an objective (Alexander, 1972). In the absence of such information not only will financial decisionmaking be faulty, but also there will be no data to present staff regarding the relative financial health of their units. Feldman (1972) pointed out that "the program budget offers a language through which the mental health agency can become more visible and comprehensible to all parties of the budget process" (p. 54).

Provided with program specific financial data, staff generally develop a significant interest in insuring a competitive edge for their program vis-à-vis other programs. A healthy competition ensues which promotes a greater degree of staff ownership of and control over their programs.

Multiplicity of Funding Sources

Within an economy of scarcity and unpredictability, the mental health administrator is well advised to rely on diverse funding sources (Silber, 1974). However, this is much easier said than done:

> Multiple financing implies a significant and complex role for the mental health executive in the area of financing. He must be an innovative and efficient manager; a long range financial planner, and a salesman familiar with the political process and possessing grantsmanship ability. (Havey, 1973, p. 119)

His clinical training and personal inclinations may make the mental health administrator reluctant to pursue funding vigorously. This reluctance will be reflected in inadequate financial planning to secure funds and unpersuasive presentations to potential funding groups. The process of "massaging the public system for mental health," Potter (1975) pointed out, entails knowing how and by whom funds are allocated and disbursed, developing personal relationships with key people in the public funding system, and aggressively seeking funds.

Contingency Planning

In the end, even the most aggressive and competent administrator may not be able to exercise sufficient influence on external funding sources. The competent administrator must take account of this possibility and plan accordingly. Contingency planning requires the administrator to maintain a balance between hoping for the best and preparing for the worst.

Human service administrators in general are far more successful in developing new programs than in curtailing or terminating services in response to declining resources. Their professional value system predisposes them to justify services on the basis of need rather than financial capacity. Nevertheless, it is the responsibility of the administrator to insure the financial stability of the mental health organization.

According to Whittington (1975), successful contingency planning requires:

1. hard data on financial trends and service productivity
2. contact with potential funding sources to assess, as accurately as possible, financing alternatives
3. input from key management in exploring all options and formulating a plan and commitment from them to its implementation
4. objective criteria based upon board policy and known to all participants
5. renegotiation of professional objectives and program priorities with the community

Information Management

The mental health administrator must make decisions based on sound management information relevant to the objectives of the organization. However, a management information system (MIS) is no magical problem solver but solely a systematic process of assembling facts so that the administrator can make intelligent decisions (Welder, 1973). And, like community mental health itself, the MIS has been overrated and oversold. Sophisticated information systems are costly; they may also be too elaborate for the organization and too little in demand (Pollock, 1974). Consequently, the administrator should carefully evaluate the information needs of his organization. Several key questions should be asked:

1. Have we first developed a manual system so that we know what information we want and that the input we have developed will produce it (Cooper, 1974)?
2. Have we defined and clarified the basic organizational goals that will be accomplished (Levy, 1970)?
3. Do we have in place the management structure to insure reliability and accuracy of input documents?
4. Are the staff persuaded to "buy into the system" (Nelson, 1973)?
5. Have we clarified our expectations to make them realistic (O'Brien, 1973)?
6. Does the system meet the criteria of client confidentiality, flexibility, and economy (Wilder and Miller, 1973)?

The decision to proceed with an MIS must be the product of extensive deliberation at all levels of staff. Holder (1970) observed that the mental health field suffers from "data gluttony and information starvation." The mental health system, he urged, needs a comprehensive program for the acquisition, dissemination, interpretation, and utilization of relevant information that can serve three major systems: external, intrasystem, and intersystem. For example, the intrasystem needs—those of the organization itself—pertain to financial management, clinical management, and planning and evaluation:

1. Financial management requirements include billing, rate setting, budget report production, and financial forecasting.
2. Clinical management requires medical and psychiatric information on clients and data on continuity of care.
3. Planning and evaluation requirements include demographic data on clients, needs assessment data, and outcome measures.

McPheeters (1970) identified five principal functions of data systems in community mental health settings:

1. assessment of the problems that are to be addressed
2. record keeping of patient treatment
3. evaluation of program effectiveness
4. development of new and improved programs
5. basic research into fundamental problems facing the system

Some very exciting progress is being made in automating clinical records. A problem oriented approach to this task promises to facilitate evaluation of treatment effectiveness. This capability is crucial in view of the demand for public accountability.

Cost-effectiveness, another aspect of public accountability, can best be measured by demonstrating the lowest unit cost possible, consistent with national standards. Staff must achieve the highest possible level of service productivity in order to reduce the unit of service cost. This can be done only in a system that routinely documents staff transactions and translates these transactions into costs. As described earlier, the availability and utilization of such data can profoundly influence staff performance.

MISs in mental health organizations run into trouble when system development and operation is assigned to research units. Line staff resent domination of the MIS by researchers, whom they believe use the data to write papers.

Most of the major problems encountered in the implementation of an MIS in fact are manpower related. The organizational readiness for an MIS has far more to do with staff preparedness than with the availability of technical or financial resources. Typical initial responses to the development of an MIS include:

1. Denial—"I really don't believe it's happening."
2. Neglect—"Maybe if I ignore it, it will go away."
3. Hostility—anger at the intrusion and refusal to comply.
4. Defensiveness—anger, with reluctant compliance.
5. Criticism—"The MIS isn't delivering what it promised."
6. Toleration—output documents are beginning to cut down on some clerical tasks.
7. Grudging acceptance—"The MIS is here to stay, so I'd better get with it."
8. Acceptance—input documents become routine and increasingly accurate.
9. Support—questions are formulated to explore further uses of the system; output documents are beginning to be used.

This process may take two to five years, depending upon various organizational factors. Because the quality and reliability of input documents begin to improve only during the later phases, implementation of the system requires tremendous patience on the part of the administrator and the MIS staff. Attempts to short-circuit the process could well undermine the reliability and utility of an MIS for a considerably longer period.

Mental health professional staff initially resent the MIS. In a field characterized by relative autonomy and dedicated to intangibles, clinicians may see an MIS as the beginning of mass production and the end of the professionalization of their services. An understanding of the real demands of public accountability may help staff appreciate that the effective implementation of an MIS may be the salvation of mental health services:

> The problem is not that mental health professionals lack decision-making skills, but they tend, by virtue of their training and credentials, to see themselves as individual entrepreneurs, who need not be involved in organizational planning

and who are not accountable for the achievement of organizational objectives. . . .

A management information system can be best developed and implemented in a mental health organization in which all workers identify with organizational objectives. This identification can only be accomplished by sound management in all areas of the organization. (Wilder and Miller, 1973, p. 136)

Staff and Structural Considerations

In human service organizations and mental health programs in particular, personnel management is organizational management and vice versa. Staff costs usually consume between 75 percent and 90 percent of the financial resources of a community mental health program. Successful personnel and organizational management requires the balancing and integration of staff and agency needs.

Personnel Management

An organization is an accumulation of individuals, each with his own personality and idiosyncracies—some hidden, others overt (Elwell, 1975). A mental health organization is further complicated by the heterogeneity of staff, including professional, paraprofessional, clerical, and administrative personnel—whose backgrounds may set them at odds (Block, 1974).

The mental health administrator must understand that he can never keep everyone happy; in fact, he will seldom keep anyone really satisfied. This represents a serious problem for the clinical administrator, who by personality and training is disposed to want and need acceptance and support from his fellow professionals (Levinson and Klerman, 1967). At the same time, once the clinician ascends to the position of administrator, the staff are no longer his colleagues but his subordinates. To maintain staff morale, the administrator must chart a course of action and implement that plan in a manner that will achieve the long-term goals of the organization.

Any decision the administrator makes may generate staff discontent. This will be particularly true of decisions involving changes that are likely to threaten the autonomy or status of particular persons or groups (Mechanic, 1973). Therefore, it is incumbent on the administrator to make decisions in a manner that will enhance not his popularity but his respect among staff. Some guidelines are suggested here.

A review of these criteria should not imply, however, that all administrative decisions require this level of attention.

Sensitivity. It is essential for staff to feel that the administrator understands their perspective on any issue. The clinical administrator can bring to bear his clinical skills of listening and empathizing, without losing the administrative decisionmaking perspective. To meet with groups of staff on specific issues helps them to know that their concerns are appreciated.

Fairness. This quality is far more important to staff in developing respect for their leader than is agreement. The administrator must demonstrate that his decisions are not based entirely on his own preferences or those of a particular subgroup of staff. The administrator's decisionmaking track record is the best indication of this quality.

Clarity. Whatever position or decision the administrator chooses, he must be explicit and direct. The staff of a mental health program are experts in human behavior. They will immediately detect uncertainty and pursue its implications. Therefore, the administrator must be clear about what a decision means before he commits himself to it.

Objectivity. In explicating his decision, the administrator must be clear about the criteria he used. Staff will demand this information. Reliance on objective and rational criteria will enhance the staff's respect for the administrator and confidence in his leadership.

Decisiveness. Clinical administrators are averse to appearing inflexible. However, flexibility has a place only in the input phase of decisionmaking. Once a decision has been announced, it must be nonnegotiable. Accordingly, any contingencies related to a decision must be communicated to staff both to permit alternative courses of action as appropriate and to protect the administrator's credibility.

Consistency. Mental health professionals are sensitive to behavioral nuances. Inconsistency on the part of the administrator exposes him to staff mistrust. Thus, the administrator sometimes will have to make decisions that run counter to his own preferences but follow the policy guidelines he has established.

Of course, the administrator is not the only decisionmaker in the organization. Therefore, he must choose staff who are respected by their coworkers and are likely to have strong opinions of their own. In addition, staff should represent various professional disciplines and clinical approaches. Staff selection is discussed in more detail later. Suffice it to say here that the administrator is only part of the decisionmaking process. The nature of a mental health organization, whose staff demand a high level of autonomy, favors horizontal decisionmaking.

There are strictly clinical decisions that are completely within the prerogative of caseworkers and other clinicians to make. Clerical staff make administrative support decisions every day. There are client support decisions that paraprofessional staff make. All of these decisions fall within the parameters of existing policy and require no review or approval. But staff must be aware of organizational policy and procedures in order to know within what parameters they are free to operate. It is the responsibility of the administrator to insure, through the organizational chain of authority, that the decisionmaking parameters are clear to all staff. Any justifiable need for deviation from existing policy should be approved at the lowest level possible (DeVito, 1974).

In his role as decisionmaker, the administrator of a mental health organization should bear several factors in mind.

1. Beware of a deputy director who frees the administrator of many an internal preoccupation but in the process separates him from staff and organizational activities. This situation is particularly risky if the deputy director is a business, management, or financial expert. The philosophy and even the personality of an organization are reflective of the chief executive officer. As noted earlier, in a mental health organization, one of the major functions of the administrator is to integrate the clinical perspective with that of management. The deputy director is not qualified to perform this critical job.

Despite the pressures on the administrator to focus on external affairs, he must be ever mindful of not abdicating the integrative role. This is not to say that responsibilities cannot be delegated; however, there is danger that as pressure mounts to deal with external funding and regulatory organizations, the administrator may, more by default than by design, neglect this important leadership function.

2. The management of professional roles is complex: "Mental health organizations are not merely formal organizations, but by their very character bring into sharp focus many of the complexities of organizations" (Mechanic, 1973, p. 143). The existence of a clear structure, with formal channels of decisionmaking and communication; a specific division of labor expressed through job descriptions; explicit policies and procedures for staff—these are the essence of a formal organization. It is important, however, that the clinical administrator be sensitive to the human and informal aspects of the mental health agency and achieve a balance between formal and informal elements (Perlman, 1975).

As I have stressed, mental health professionals subscribe to values, inherent in their professional training, that reinforce autonomy and independence (Ryan, 1974). Their negative reaction to structure is more unconscious than deliberate and often takes the form of pseudo-egalitarianism.

Unlike more traditional hospital settings, mental health workers in community mental health centers are testing new relationships relative to clients and professionals, and since such roles are frequently not clearly defined, each of the professional groups attempts to stake out its work territory relative to other groups, new forms of cooperation, and new definitions of its scope of work autonomy and authority. (Mechanic, 1973, p. 145)

The task of the mental health administrator is to guide the construction and implementation of staff roles so as to achieve the most effective mix of skills in a manner that insures clarity, responsibility, and accountability.

3. The tension between organizational constraints and professional autonomy may also give rise to elitist groups (Mechanic, 1973). While this response may be found among any one of the mental health disciplines, it is most often ascribed to psychiatrists. The elitism and dominance of physicians in hospitals is well known. The interdisciplinary nature of the mental health organization, however, precludes acceptance of this model.

Cohen (1975) described the changing status of psychiatrists in community mental health organizations and Beigel (1975) acknowledged their loss of preeminence. My experience suggests that psychiatric staff function most productively and effectively in a mental health organization when they provide services on a contractual basis, rather than as employees.

Middle Management

A middle management team serves both as the major source of input to the administrator for decisionmaking and as the primary vehicle for the implementation of decisions. In the former role, middle managers are expected to reflect not only their own but also their staff's viewpoints. With respect to the latter role, once a decision has been made, they are expected to implement it vigorously, whatever their opinion of its merits.

Herein lies the dilemma for the middle manager. The input function is comfortable and rewarding, for middle management typically values its role in influencing policy. Moreover, this function enables middle managers to be advocates for the profession, program, or geographical region they represent. The discomfort arises when they must implement a decision that they did not support or that their staff are not likely to welcome. This creates a conflict between their formal organizational role and their informal role as staff representative. To implement unpopular decisions with the perspective of the decisionmaker, the middle administrator may jeopardize the support and acceptance of his subgroup. Therefore, he is likely to implement the decision reluctantly and, perhaps, ineffectively, thereby preserving his position with line staff.

Just as the clinician must surrender collegiality when he assumes the administrator's position, so must the middle manager circumscribe his collegiality with his staff if he is to perform effectively. The plight of the middle manager is just beginning to attract attention in mental health administration training programs. This area requires substantial study and examination. Since social workers constitute a large segment of mental health middle management, social work schools should give this issue top priority.

The chain of administration will be only as effective as its weakest link. For an administration, including top and middle management, to be sensitive, fair, clear, objective, decisive, and consistent, middle managers must shift their primary loyalty to, and must identify closely with, the administrative team. If this transition is to be successful, the administrator must assist middle management by insuring that the loss of line staff support will be compensated by administrative support.

Team building can be facilitated by periodic retreat sessions in which middle management staff are able to deal with weighty administrative policy decisions within an environment of group support; staff development opportunities that focus on enhancing communication, building trust, and fostering team cohesion; and administrative training for middle management. The chief executive must serve as a role model for middle management and relate to them in the same manner that they must relate to their staff. Each group must select from its constituency various persons among whom it can distribute tasks and privileges and from whom it can seek information and advice (Mechanic, 1973).

Two major principles are useful to the administrator in building a middle management team:

1. He must be open and honest with respect to how much and what type of authority he is willing to share vis-à-vis the decisionmaking process.
2. The administrator must specify clearly which areas are not negotiable by virtue of external regulations, existing board policy, or the chief executive's own criteria (Blankenship, 1972).

The Paradox of the Mental Health Organization

The typical mental health organization is not nonprofit, but antiprofit. Federal regulations on deficit financing require that the organization not accumulate a surplus. This constraint not only prevents the oganization from developing a minimal degree of financial security but also creates a climate of uncertainty and austerity and a demand for high productivity in an industry that deals in intangibles.

Strategies for achieving high productivity were discussed earlier. What is important to note here is that such strategies will quickly reach a point of diminishing returns unless management is able to provide positive reinforcement, in the form of a reward system, for staff efforts. Yet, the same fiscal constraints that require high levels of productivity for financial stability severely restrict the implementation of an appropriate and meaningful reward system. While job security is a powerful incentive, its effect may be short-lived in the absence of salary increases, professional development opportunities, and an organizational climate of security, predictability, and professional support.

Recruitment

The selection of staff is the most important first step in personnel management. For in the selection process, the chemistry of the organization is established, for better or for worse. With the recruitment of professional staff in particular, it is essential in advance to define selection criteria in relationship to general organizational and program goals. The Equal Employment Opportunity Act has resulted in an upgrading of the recruitment process. Today, procedures are documented, consistent, and equitable. However, these requirements can be circumvented unless administration makes it clear that they benefit the organization.

Evaluation

Human service agencies tend to evaluate professional staff in a superficial way. Staff resistance to evaluation as an intrusion upon their autonomy encourages assessments aimed only at meeting personnel policy requirements and qualifying staff for salary increases. It is a disservice to staff, clients, and the community for administration to settle for anything less than a thorough assessment of clinical staff performance in the areas of productivity, competence, relationships with colleagues and supervisors, responsiveness to clients, service to the organization, and overall maturity of judgment.

Obviously, the most difficult area to evaluate is clinical competence, and this, for the most part, has been seriously neglected. The implementation of quality assurance programs, particularly peer review, has provided a very effective mechanism for organizations to evaluate the clinical performance of staff.

One of the major objectives in human service agencies must be to tie meaningful evaluation to specific rewards in the form of salary increases, educational opportunities, and so on. This approach motivates staff and benefits both the agency and the community it serves.

Supervision

In the multidisciplinary setting of a mental health organization, supervision is likely to be provided by a member of another discipline, to include both clinical and administrative functions, and to constitute an integral part of a quality assurance program. Furthermore, as mental health programs struggle to maximize direct services, individual supervision has given way to more cost-effective group approaches. This shift will involve a substantial adjustment for social workers, who may be accustomed to individual supervision by a social work colleague. However, the Academy of Certified Social Workers requires that new graduates receive two years of MSW supervision. The candidate for employment should clarify his expectations and insure that they will be met by the mental health agency.

Termination

The literature has given little attention to the administrative process of involuntary termination. Nevertheless, nonproductive, dysfunctional, or incompetent staff cannot be retained. Termination may also be necessitated by organizational changes or budget cutbacks.

One of the major administrative weaknesses of the clinical administrator is the inability to terminate staff who are ineffective or inappropriate but want to stay within the organization. Therapeutic values influence the administrator to protect the staff member and his family from the stresses of termination. This, in the end, does a disservice to all: it leaves the staff member in the uncomfortable position of living with failure and the administration in the awkward position of being inconsistent. The usual result of this course of action is the gradual deterioration of the staff person, his loss of respect among colleagues, the development of a hostile and dependent relationship with the administrator, and an eventual, more destructive termination. Overall staff morale is also adversely affected by such a prolonged tense situation.

It is far more compassionate and therapeutic, in fact, for the administrator to deal directly and honestly with a staff member whose continued participation in the organization is inappropriate. Staff also deserve assistance in finding a position in another organization. A constructive outplacement process should consist of a thorough evaluation that identifies specific goals toward which to work and a time limit for their achievement; close supervision of problem areas; a limited time opportunity to seek other employment either within the organization at a lower, more appropriate level or in another organization; financial provisions, including separation pay or paid leave; assistance in contacting other organizations; supportive but honest references to potential employers; and a decision to terminate based upon inability or unwillingness to achieve the specified goals.

Interorganizational Diplomacy

The health field and organizational theorists (Levine and White, 1963) seem to have rediscovered something that early social work leaders took for granted, the importance of relationships between organizations. Without explicating theories of interorganizational dynamics, early social workers nevertheless concentrated on the relationships among components of the social welfare system—public welfare, courts, employment services, medical services—and their coordination in the interest of the client.

Because social workers and, subsequently, other professionals also took these relationships for granted, they did not study the factors that distinguish between arrangements that work well and those that do not. The prevailing assumption was that interagency relationships succeeded because administrators wanted to cooperate in the interests of clients.

The community mental health program, perhaps more than any other human service movement, depends on a highly effective network of cooperating agencies. The public laws that mandated the provision of twelve services made it virtually impossible for any one center to function well without one or more affiliates. Yet the technology of interorganizational activity is still primitive.

One of the major responsibilities of the mental health administrator is to negotiate with other organizations to arrange the resources necessary to his agency—funds, staff, clients, political support, etc. The typical mental health administrator, however, lacks special training in both intraorganizational and interorganizational leadership. The latter requires shrewdness, tact, forcefulness, and flexibility. Yet the same clinical administrator who approaches internal management from a social work orientation also tends to follow a therapeutic model in dealing with other organizations.

Most seasoned administrators know, and research shows that coordination between human service agencies exists when they face a common threat, when one is clearly dominant, or when one stands to benefit disproportionately from the interaction:

> The expressed motivation for and against interorganizational relationships are political rather than social. Although the administrators enunciated the socially desirable reponse of "improved services," as motivating their interagency activity, the more basic motivation was reflected in responses associated with protection of domain, authority and power. Decisions with respect to interorganizational relationships appear therefore to be made more on the basis of gains in power and domain rather than on the betterment of mankind. (Kane, 1972, p. 85)

Any strategy for developing cooperative agreements between mental health settings must recognize the political dynamics of the enterprise. In a recent article (Kane, 1980), I outlined such a strategy:

1. the predisposition of the parties for the development of a joint venture
2. the development of a negotiating mechanism
3. the establishment of a negotiation process

Successful interorganizational activity requires mutual identification of a basic organizational need and recognition that a specific arrangement will meet that organizational need for each party. In the absence of a clear indication that the organization (or the administrator) will benefit from the transaction, there is no real incentive for proceeding (Long, 1974).

In his analysis of interorganizational relations, O'Brien (1973) distinguished between relationships among organizations that are mandated by law and those that are strictly voluntary and amenable to interorganizational negotiations. In either case, the administrator must thoroughly diagnose his own interorganizational capabilities. O'Brien listed specific steps that the administrator should follow:

1. identify the boundary-spanning personnel within his own organization and the organizational constituents with whom they deal
2. assess the rewards and costs of the voluntary exchange relationship from the perspective of his own organization, as well as of the other
3. assess areas of disagreement and consensus in organizational domain and prestige and note the pattern of informal relationships
4. maintain open communications between himself and other key boundary-spanning personnel
5. identify areas of potential intervention either by third parties or by the participants themselves to increase the predictability of the organizational environment
6. attempt to formulate and communicate to staff information on the relationship between their own organization and others
7. facilitate the opening of organizational boundaries to new interorganizational liaisons at all levels

Assuming that there is an identifiable need and "a converging of interests" (Aram, 1974), the administrator must initiate a negotiations process to identify problems and issues that must be confronted. Specifically, the negotiating mechanism should be characterized by three features.

1. Clarification of negotiable and nonnegotiable items. The failure to specify nonnegotiable issues can lead the parties into polarized positions, which could jeopardize the entire venture.

2. Identification of external constraints. As O'Brien (1973) pointed out, mandated relationships and/or requirements will significantly limit the flexibility of the process and must be mutually acknowledged.

3. Establishment of priorities. It is crucial that each organization identify the priority needs that must be met through the negotiation process.

Both parties must distinguish between needs and wants. The ability of the negotiating agencies to document their needs in such a way that they become mutual objectives rather than unilateral pursuits can transform a win-lose situation into a win-win process.

The Negotiating Process

A serious mistake occurs when negotiations are pursued primarily by two chief executives. For an interorganizational arrangement to be effective over time, all appropriate levels of the organization—board, administration, and clinical staff—must participate in order to insure that commitment to, and support for, the end product is evenly distributed down the line.

Board members meet a major organizational need in advocating organizational interests with opinion leaders and decisionmakers in other organizations and in the community. Board members who themselves have a measure of power and influence in the larger society can achieve interorganizational objectives that may well be beyond the capacity of the mental health agency administrator.

At the other extreme, line staff constantly function at organizational boundaries with line staff of other organizations in the delivery of services. The credibility and influence promoted by competent staff and effective services can easily be underestimated by the administrator in his effort to enhance relationships with the external environment.

Implications for Social Work

The conceptual underpinnings of interorganizational relations are rooted in open systems theory, which emphasizes that an organization in the process of staying afloat and striving to achieve its goals draws resources from the environment that are the raw material for production (Perlmutter, 1974). For community mental health programs, this translates into the need to develop a care giving network that includes other human service agencies and individual community caretakers—i.e., physicians, clergy, and teachers (Schulberg, 1970).

While formal administrative negotiations are likely to take place at the senior management level, direct service staff are more likely to determine in the end whether interorganizational arrangements succeed or fail, and social workers in particular are in a strategic position to influence outcome (Ivey, 1970).

Social workers occupy key positions both in middle management and at the service boundaries of mental health organizations (Kane, 1972). The question remains as to whether and to what extent social workers are willing and able to capitalize on their positions in the community mental health system to achieve goals that have been identified by the profession. These goals include the provision of comprehensive services available as needed to individuals and groups. The type of continuity and coordination of services indicated by the concept of comprehensiveness obviously cannot be achieved without effective interorganizational arrangements.

If social workers are to serve as links in insuring these arrangements, they must be trained in interorganizational dynamics. In recent years the profession has made a substantial contribution to the conceptual base of social work practice. Increased attention to such social science tools as organizational theory, systems theory, and power concepts may well enable social workers to achieve the full potential of their role as interorganizational linkages in comprehensive human service systems.

Citizen Participation

In the past twenty years consumer activism has burgeoned. Although social work traditionally has advocated self-determination, community involvement, and mobilization of local resources, including indigenous leaders, the community mental health movement of the 1960s gave new life to this orientation.

Citizen participation, however, means different things to different people. Community participation may be viewed in several contexts: volunteers, consumers, board members, and organization members (Kaplan, 1973).

The nature of citizen participation also varies with its objective:

1. Organizational—to set agency policy: for "Through the participation of community groups in the identification of problems, issues and service goals, it is hoped that agency programs gain more community legitimacy" (Kaplan, 1973, p. 212).
2. Political—to bring about a realignment of power within the community in favor of community interests (mental health) that have been underserved in the past and to achieve some measure of social change.

A variety of community board models exists. Their authority ranges from complete control to a purely advisory role. While all these models are used in mental health organizations, the federal mandate envisions the greatest possible level of community control:

Support for local community control and citizen participation in the development, delivery and evaluation of mental health services continues to be a central component of federal legislation. That encouragement is based on the assumption that direct citizen involvement in the administration and monitoring of mental health services is likely to produce improved program accountability and responsiveness, as well as qualitative, equitable care to all sectors of the community. (National Institute of Mental Health, 1978, p. iii)

Board Selection

The federal establishment has tended to encourage citizen participation as an end in itself rather than as a strategy for accomplishing organizational objectives (Kane, 1975). The myth reflected in this assumption is that community representation per se will insure effective governance. This has not proven to be the case, and the federal government has retreated somewhat from its earlier position.

The constitution of a board should reflect the phase of organizational development and the major organizational goals. Moreover, research has shown that the most active board participants are people optimistic about helping mentally ill and emotionally distressed clients and dedicated to the concept of citizen participation (Jenry, 1973). Therefore, the key criteria for selection of board members should relate to these two factors rather than stress representativeness.

If citizen participation is viewed as a strategy for achieving organizational objectives, the board must both have the skills and competence to carry out its major functions and share the values of the communities the organization serves.

Board Functions

The governing body has ten major functions:

1. legal—secure and maintain the legal corporate existence of the ogranization
2. needs assessment—determine service delivery priorities through an assessment of area needs
3. planning for board operations—establish the goals and objectives of the organization and evaluate the level of achievement of the objectives
4. policymaking—determine (in collaboration with the administrator) the policies that will guide the organization
5. fiscal management—establishment of all fiscal policies, budget development and approval, and fundraising
6. public relations—interpret the organization to the community
7. advocacy—for both the community's and the organization's interests

8. community coordination—promote positive relations and working relationships with other community bodies
9. evaluation—of the center's programs, procedures, and policies, as well as of the board's performance
10. selecting an executive director—to whom the board will delegate full authority and responsibility for operating the center

No one of these board functions can be effectively performed without close cooperation between the board and the executive. The director has the responsibility to provide the board with the data necessary to assure them that the organization's activities and services are being carried out within the policies set down by the board.

Responsibilities of the Executive Director

The executive functions as the chief officer of the board. As such, he has five major tasks to carry out: (1) planning the implementation of board policy, (2) organizing all elements of the center to implement policy, (3) mobilizing and motivating personnel to implement policy, (4) controlling the implementation of policy, and (5) evaluating the implementation of policy.

Major problems can arise between the board and its executive when the line between policy development and policy implementation is unclear. Conflicts may be precipitated by an executive who attempts to encroach on the policymaking authority of the board or otherwise undermine the board's authority. Conflict can arise as well when the board inappropriately intrudes into the arena of administration:

> The crux of the problem [is] the inability to distinguish between policy-making and administrative issues—between decisions politically feasible for community representatives and those which absolutely [require] the technical competence of professional program administration. (National Institute of Mental Health, 1978, p. 70)

Carver (1979) pointed out that while the board has the authority of determine how far into the policymaking-implementation continuum it wishes to reach, once it has defined its position it must be consistent about not going beyond that point.

The quality of the relationship between the board and the executive director is the single greatest determinant of the management effectiveness of the organization. The burden is on both the administrator and the board constantly to work at achieving and maintaining the best possible combination of the skills and contributions that each has to offer.

Board Education and Training

An effective way to manage the power dynamic is the implementation of training programs which are designed to increase the competence of the board to exercise their legitimate role and overtly to cede to them greater control over the organization. An educational process that assists the board in distinguishing between policymaking and policy implementation; clarifies the role and functions of the board vis-à-vis those of the administration; and uncovers underlying conflicts over power will help stabilize the board-executive relationship.

Some administrators discourage training programs for board members as a means of maintaining control:

> Analyses of governing Boards consistently find that with adequate initial training and continued support, Boards can contribute significantly to the effectiveness of a center's operations, but unfortunately the commitment of the administration to the Board training and support is usually weak or totally absent. (National Institute of Mental Health, 1978, p. 56)

An uninformed and incompetent board is, however, far more damaging to the organization and the administrator's performance than one that is properly equipped to meet its responsibilities.

Community Development

For a board to serve as an effective change agent, it must have the capacity to gain the support of prominent local business persons and officials, as well as community leaders. The administrator, in turn, must be knowledgeable about community organization and group processes. The development and management of community support is embedded in the traditional practice of social work, and the community organization concepts and methodology of social work are directly applicable to the effective utilization of community boards in the achievement of all their major functions. The historic commitment of the social work profession to citizen participation and client self-determination can sustain the mental health administrator in the difficult job of attracting and keeping the community's interest in the agency's fortunes.

A mental health program is, by its very nature, a change agent that threatens the community status quo: "One of the greatest obstacles that has interrupted the goal of the CMHC Act has been the hostility of the community against accepting the mentally ill living in the community" (National Institute of Mental Health, 1978, p. 24). To dissipate this hostility and develop community support demands from both board and administrator the best that each has to offer.

Issues and Trends

The health and human services are being held to an unprecedented level of accountability. Costs and treatment outcomes must be scrutinized not only by funding sources but also by agency administrators if they are to fulfill their federal mandate. Evaluation, however, has to be followed up by action—reallocation of resources, provision of new services, termination of incompetent staff, fundraising, and so on. Yet public program administrators are particularly reluctant to be guided by cost-benefit analysis:

> Service institutions are not want oriented; they are need oriented. By definition they are concerned with "good works" and with "social" or "moral" contributions rather than with returns and benefits. The social worker will always believe that the very failure of her effort to get a family off welfare proves that more effort and more money are needed. She cannot accept that her failure—continuous and total over half a century—means that she had better stop what she is so valiantly failing in. (Drucker, 1980, p. 44)

The fiscal climate of the 1980s is likely to make mental health administrators acutely sensitive to balance-sheet considerations.

Marketing

The new emphasis on productivity in service occupations calls for a more entrepreneurial approach to the development, packaging, and delivery of health and human services. Proven techniques from private industry for the promotion and marketing of consumer goods may be applicable to mental health (Kane, 1980).

Performance Contracts

Most public funds for human services will be provided through the vehicle of performance contracts, which may be subject to competitive bidding. Mental health agencies may have to compete with other health and human service organizations to secure or maintain federal, state, or local financial support.

The number of units of service to be provided will be specified by program, and by client population, with emphasis on high-risk groups—the elderly, chronic patients, and minorities—who are also least able to pay for services. Performance contracts will also specify individual staff responsibilities, as well as benefits to be gained through successful performance.

Staff Incentive Programs

Incentive programs can maximize staff investment in the service goals of the organization. Revenue sharing may be incorporated into staff incentive programs, along with flexible policies on private practice and flexible work schedules.

Planning

Successful planning requires a shift away from needs assessment to predict future utilization of services to a marketing research approach that can predict wants. This shift is dictated by the major change that will take place as mental health organizations move from a public service model based on declining public funding to an entrepreneurial model based on client fees and third-party payments. Effective planning aimed at securing federal resources also must address the requirements of the 1980 Mental Health Systems Act, which mandated new approaches to service development and new service areas and identified high-priority target populations.

Whatever the potential benefits of capitalizing on federal resources available through the Mental Health Systems Act, exclusive dependence or any one source of funds—particularly public taxes—is dangerous. Long-term stability depends on the mental health agency's ability to diversify its services, clients, and sources of revenue.

Conflicts

The shift to a more entrepreneurial approach in the administration of mental health services will bring to the surface major value conflicts for the social worker, who is committed both to serving high-risk clients who cannot pay for services and insuring the financial stability of the organization. These value conflicts must, in the end, be resolved at the governance board level but will nevertheless require tremendous soul searching on the part of the staff and the mental health administrator. Current legislation has aggravated this conflict by giving high priority to nonpaying clients and low priority to supporting such services. Achieving a creative balance in this area may well be the greatest challenge to the mental health administrator of the future.

REFERENCES

ALEXANDER, J. B., and MESSAL, J. L. "The Planning-Programming-Budgeting System in the Mental Health Field." *Hospital and Community Psychiatry* 1972, *23*(12):357–361.

ANDRE, P., KANE, T. J., and MEYER, J., Jr. "Economic Assessment: A Model." *Administration in Mental Health* 1978, *6*(winter):107–119.

ARAM, J. D., and STRATTEN, W. E. "The Development of Interagency Cooperation." *Social Service Review* 1974, *48*(3):12–21.

AUSTIN, M. "Evaluating the Training of Mental Health Administrators." *Administration in Mental Health* 1975, (winter):57–67.

AU YEURY, B. "A Study of Citizen Participation in Community Mental Health Centers." *Dissertation Abstracts International* 1973, no. 73-21339.

BAKER, F. "Planning and the Environment of a Community Mental Health Center." *Psychiatric Quarterly* 1972, *46*(1):95–108.

BEIGEL, A. "The Psychiatrist-Administrator: Odd Man Out?" *Community Mental Health Journal* 1975, *11*(2):129–135.

BINDMAN, A. J. "The Psychologist as a Mental Health Administrator." *Professional Psychology* 1970, *1*(5):445–447.

BLANKERSHIP, R. L. "The Emerging Organization of a Community Mental Health Center." *Dissertation Abstracts International* 1972, no. 72-12091.

BLOCK, W. E. "The Study of Attitudes about Mental Health in the Community Mental Health Center." *Community Mental Health Journal* 1974, *10*(2):216–220.

BURGESS, J. "Who Has the Administrative Skills in Mental Health?" *Public Administration Review* 1974, *33*(2):164–167.

BURKE, E. M. "Planning for Bellak's Third Revolution." *Community Mental Health Journal* 1969, *5*(3):256–263.

CARVER, J. "Community Participation: How to Turn It Around; Mistakes, Myths, and Thoughts About." Manuscript, 1979.

COHEN, J. "Themes of Leadership." In G. Magner (ed.), *Leadership Training in Mental Health.* New York: National Association of Social Workers, 1970.

COHEN, R. E. "New Career Models for Future Psychiatrists." In L. Bellack and H. H. Barten (eds.), *Progress in Community Mental Health,* vol. 3. New York: Brunner Mazel, 1975.

COOPER, E. M. *Guidelines for a Minimum Statistical and Accounting System for Community Mental Health Centers.* DHEW pub. no. (ADM) 74-14. Washington, D.C.: U.S. Government Printing Office, 1974.

CRAWFORD, J. L., MORGAN, D. W., and GIANTURO, D. T. (eds.). *Progress in Mental Health Information Systems.* Cambridge: Ballinger, 1975.

CROWN, L. E. "Meaningful Consumer Participation—A Challenge to the Social Agency Administration." In H. A. Schatz (ed.), *Social Work Administration.* New York: Council on Social Work Education, 1970.

DESOLE, D., SINGER, P., and SWIETNICKI, E. "A Project That Failed." In L. Duhl and R. L. Leopold (eds.), *Mental Health and Urban Social Policy: A Casebook of Community Action.* San Francisco: Jossey-Bass, 1968.

DEVITO, R. A. "The Supervisory Bypass: A Symptom of Organizational Anxiety." *Hospital and Community Psychiatry* 1974, *25*(11):724–725.

DIAMOND, H. and SANTORE, A. "Basic Tasks in Developing a Community Mental Health Center." *Hospital and Community Psychiatry* 1974, *25*(4):232–235.

DOLGOFF, T. "Power, Conflict, and Structure in Mental Health Organizations: A General Systems Analysis." *Administration in Mental Health* 1972 (winter): 12–21.

DRUCKER, P. F. *Management: Tasks, Responsibilities, Practices.* New York: Harper & Row, 1973.

ELWELL, R. N. "What the Administrator Needs to Know about the Clinician; What the Clinician Needs to Know about the Administrator: Perceptions and Problems." In R. Agranoff and A. Dykstra, Jr. (eds.), *Mental Health in Transition.* Lansing, Mich.: Association of Mental Health Administrators, 1975.

FELDMAN, S. (ed.). *The Administration of Mental Health Services.* Springfield, Ill.: Thomas, 1973.

——. "Budgeting and Behavior." In S. Feldman (ed.), *The Administration of Mental Health Services.* Springfield, Ill.: Thomas, 1973.

——. "Convergence and Conflict: The Mental Health Professional in Government." *Public Administration Review* 1978, *38*(2):139–144. (a)

——. "Promises, Promises or Community Mental Health Services and Training: Ships That Pass in the Night." *Community Mental Health Journal* 1978, 14(2):83–91. (b)

——. "Leadership in Mental Health: Changing the Guard for the 1980's." Eugene Hargrave Lecture Series, Raleigh, North Carolina, October 1979.

HAVEY, E. C. "Financing Mental Health Services." In S. Feldman (ed.), *The Administration of Mental Health Services.* Springfield, Ill.: Thomas, 1973.

HOLDER, H. D. "Evaluation Methods and Dynamics in Program Planning." In C. R. Wurster (ed.), *Statistics in Mental Health Programs.* Washington, D.C.: National Clearinghouse for Mental Health Information, 1970.

HOWELL, J. P. "The Characteristics of Administration and the Effectiveness of Community Mental Health Centers." *Administration in Mental Health* 1976, *3*(spring):125–132.

HUTCHESON, B. R., and KRAUSE, E. A. "Systems Analysis and Mental Health Services." *Community Mental Health Journal* 1969, *5*(1):29–45.

IVEY, A. E., and HINKLE, J. E. "A Study in Role Theory: Liaison between Social Agencies." *Community Mental Health Journal* 1970, *6*(1):63–68.

KANE, T. J. "Social Science Concepts in Mental Health Planning." Manuscript, Catholic University, Washington, D.C., 1970.

——. "A Study of the Interorganizational Relationship between Community Mental Health Centers and Family Service Agencies." Ph.D. dissertation, Catholic University, Washington, D.C., 1972.

——. "Community Mental Health Center Cooperative Agreements: A Case of Shotgun Weddings." *Administration in Mental Health* 1980, *8*(winter):124–132.

——. "Marketing Strategies in Community Mental Health Centers." Demonstration project proposal submitted to the National Institute of Mental Health, 1980.

——, and MEYER, J., JR. "Citizen Participation in Mental Health: Myth or Strategy." *Administration in Mental Health* 1975 (spring):29–34.

KAPLAN, S. "Community Participation" In S. Feldman (ed.), *The Administration of Mental Health Services.* Springfield, Ill.: Thomas, 1973.

KOLB, L. C. "Who Should Administer Psychiatric Facilities." *Hospital and Community Psychiatry* 1969, *20*(6)170–173.

LEVIN, R. A. "Consumer Participation in Planning and Evaluation of Mental Health Services." *Social Work* 1970, *15*(2):41–46.

LEVINSON, D. J., and KLERMAN, G. L. "The Clinician-Executive: Some Problematic Issues for the Psychiatrist in Mental Health Organizations." *Psychiatry* 1967, *30*(1):3–15.

———. "The Clinician-Executive Revisited." *Administration in Mental Health* 1972 (winter):64–67.

LEVY, A. H., BAKER, R. L., JR., and CARRICK, J. M. "Electronic Information Programs: An Inhospital System." *Hospital and Community Psychiatry* 1970, *21*(1):7–10.

LITTLESTONE, R. "Planning in Mental Health." In S. Feldman (ed.), *The Administration of Mental Health Services.* Springfield, Ill.: Thomas, 1973.

LONG, N. "A Model for Coordinating Human Services." *Administration in Mental Health* 1974 (summer):21–27.

MACLEOD, R. K. "Program Budgeting Works in Nonprofit Institutions." *Harvard Business Review* 1971, *49*(5):46–56.

MALOOF, B. "Peculiarities of Human Service Bureaucracies." *Administration in Mental Health* 1975, *3*(fall):21–26.

MARVALD, M. "An Indictment of the Community Mental Health Centers Act: Caveat Emptor." *Hospital and Community Psychiatry* 1971, *22*(3):79–83.

MECHANIC, D. "The Sociology of Organizations." In S. Feldman (ed.), *The Administration of Mental Health Services.* Springfield, Ill.: Thomas, 1973.

McPHEETERS, H. S. "Data Systems and Their Application to Current Mental Health Programs." In C. R. Wurster (ed.), *Statistics in Mental Health Programs.* Washington, D.C.: National Clearinghouse for Mental Health, 1970.

National Institute of Mental Health. *Citizen Participation in Community Mental Health Centers.* Washington, D.C.: U.S. Department of Health, Education, and Welfare, 1978.

———. *Citizen Orientation Manual.* Washington, D.C.: Citizen Participation Branch, Supt. of Documents, 1979.

NELSON, C., and MORGAN, L. "The Information Systems of a Community Mental Health Center." *Administration in Mental Health* 1973 (fall):26–38.

O'BRIEN, G. M. "Information Utilization in Human Service Management: The Decision Support System Approach." Paper given at the National Conference on Social Welfare, Atlantic City, May 1973.

———. "Interorganizational Relations." In S. Feldman (ed.), *The Administration of Mental Health Services.* Springfield, Ill.: Thomas 1973.

PERLAM, B., and TORNATSKY, L. G. "Organizational Perspectives on Community Mental Health Centers." *Administration in Mental Health* 1975, *3*(fall):27–31.

PERLMUTTER, F., HEINEMANN, S., and YUDIN, L. W. "Public Welfare Clients and Community Mental Health Centers." *Public Welfare* 1974, *32*(2):29–32.

POLLACK, E. S., WINDLE, C. D., and WURSTER, C. R. "Psychiatric Information Systems: An Historical Perspective." In J. Crawford (ed.), *Progress in Mental Health Information Systems.* Cambridge: Ballinger, 1974.

POTTER, R. F. "Massaging the Public System for Mental Health Funding." In R. Agranoff and A. Dykstra, Jr. (eds.), *Mental Health in Transition.* Lansing, Mich.: Association of Mental Health Administrators, 1975.

RUTMAN, I. S., and EGAN, K. L. *The Future Role of State Mental Hospitals: A National Survey of Planning and Program Trends.* Philadelphia: Horizon House for Research and Development, n.d.

RYAN, M. "Managing Mental Health Professionals: An Alternative Future." *Administration in Mental Health* 1974 (summer):68–73.

SCHATZ, H. A. (ed.). *Social Work Administration: A Resource Book.* New York: Council on Social Work Education, 1970.

SCHULBERG, H. C., and BAKER, F. "The Caregiving System in Community Mental Health Programs: An Application of Open-Systems Theory." *Community Mental Health Journal* 1970, 6(6):437–446.

SCHWARTZ, E. E. "Some Views on the Study of Social Welfare Administration." In H. A. Shatz (ed.), *Social Work Administration: A Resource Book.* New York: Council on Social Work Education, 1970.

SCOBIE, R. S. *Social Planning in the Community Context: Six Principles for Planners.* Waltham, Mass.: Florence Heller Graduate School for Advanced Studies in Social Welfare, Brandeis University, 1971.

SILBER, S. "Strategies for Developing Multisource Funding for Community Mental Health Centers." *Hospital and Community Psychiatry* 1974, 25(4):221–225.

SILVERS, J. B., and PRAHALAD, C. K. *Financial Management of Community Institutions.* New York: Wiley, 1974.

STEGER, J. A., WOODHOUSE, R., and GOOCEY, R. "The Clinical Manager: Performance and Management Characteristics. *Administration in Mental Health* 1973 (fall):76–81.

WAGNER, B., BREITMEYER, R. G., and BOTTUM, G. "Administrative Problem Solving and the Mental Health Professional." *Professional Psychology* 1975, 6(1):55–60.

WHITTINGTON, H. G. "Survival Strategies for Community Mental Health Centers." In L. Bellack and H. H. Barton (eds.), *Progress in Community Mental Health,* vol. 3. New York: Brunner/Mazel, 1975.

WILDER, J. F., and MILLER, S. "Management Information." In S. Feldman (ed.), *The Administration of Mental Health Services.* Springfield, Ill.: Thomas, 1973.

YOLLES, S. F. "The Importance of Administration in Mental Health." *Administration in Mental Health* 1975, 3(fall):43–50.

CHAPTER 7

Planning

Louis E. DeMoll

PRIOR TO World War II, there was little evidence of a national commitment to mental health planning. Most planning efforts were related to improving physical facilities of state mental hospitals or responding to criticisms of occasional reform efforts to enhance the care of the mentally ill. Planning for mental health programs became more formal with the passage of the National Mental Health Act of 1946 (P.L. 79–487). Shocked by the realization that more than one million young men had been rejected for military service in World War II because of psychiatric disabilities, with thousands of others succumbing to emotional illnesses while on active duty, Congress responded with a program to improve the mental health of the general population (U.S. Congress, 1945). In the following year, funds were appropriated to implement the goals of the landmark legislation. To achieve the long-range aims of Congress, the following programs were launched under P.L. 79–487:

1. research—to seek ways to prevent mental disability
2. training—to develop an adequate supply of manpower in all mental health disciplines
3. formula grants to states—to assist states in developing community mental health services, conducting demonstration projects, and providing inservice training for state and local personnel

The National Mental Health Act also established the National Institute of Mental Health as a formal part of the nation's health system. Advisory committees were authorized to recommend to the federal government procedures for monitoring the country's mental health service delivery system and for developing long-term planning strategies. Planning in mental health received a significant stimulus when the National Institute of Mental Health announced that the states would have to submit a plan for the utilization of the formula grant funds that were available for community mental health services. Because of this requirement, state mental health staff began a systematic review of needs; priorities were established; and program strategies to meet human service needs were designed and incorporated into the annual mental health plan.

Social workers made important contributions to the early efforts of the Community Services Branch of the National Institute of Mental Health to plan and develop a mental health program at the national level. Lamson (1954) underscored the strategic value of social workers in describing their pioneering role in providing consultative services to states in developing and coordinating state planning efforts with national planning goals. The Community Services Branch social work consultants encouraged states to develop plans that would address their unique needs rather than follow a uniform format.

The decade after the founding of the National Institute of Mental Health saw significant advances in manpower training, program development, community practice, and research. Unfortunately, state hospitals reaped few of these benefits.

Planning received another stimulus in 1955 with the enactment of the Mental Health Study Act (P.L. 84–182). Discouraged by increasing state hospital populations, the Congress called for a reevaluation of the human problems associated with mental illness. The House and Senate passed a joint resolution authorizing a sweeping study of the problems of mental illness and the resources available for meeting these problems. The Joint Commission on Mental Illness and Health was formed to implement the congressional mandate (Joint Commission on Mental Illness and Health, 1961).

After a five-year period of study, the commission's report to Congress, *Action for Mental Health,* was forwarded to President John F. Kennedy. In 1962, Congress provided funds to the National Institute of Mental Health to implement the recommendations of the commission. The funds were used to assist the states in developing comprehensive mental health plans. Congress reasoned that a system of planning grants would accelerate the job of carrying out the far-reaching recommendations of the commission report (U.S. Congress, 1962). In many states the planning grants provided the first opportunity for mental health personnel from community and state institutional programs to work together to study the population's total mental health needs.

In February 1963, President Kennedy sent his recommendations to Congress. The proposals had been developed from the commission report. This occasion was the first time in the nation's history that a president delivered a special message to Congress on mental health and mental retardation. President Kennedy's call for a "bold, new approach" resulted in passage of the Community Mental Health Centers Construction Act of 1963 (P.L. 88-164). Through this legislation, the National Institute of Mental Health began to encourage the development of community oriented plans that stressed a participatory process of planning.

Subsequent federal laws have influenced the direction of mental health planning. The National Health Planning and Resources Development Act of 1974 (P.L. 93-641) was signed into law in January 1975. This legislation unveiled new requirements for planning. It stipulated that states must develop a certificate of need program and establish health service areas. The law further required each state to prepare and revise annually a state health plan.

In states with a separate mental health authority and health department, there has been some mild confusion because of the overlap of authority under federal law. Usually the state health department has responsibility for health planning under the National Health Planning and Resources Development Act, while the state mental health agency (the mental health authority) is responsible for mental health planning through the authority of other federal legislation.

Adding to the complexity of federal legislation on mental health planning is the Special Health Revenue Sharing Act of 1975 (P.L. 94-63). This law was designed to strengthen mental health planning at the state level and to encourage effective planning for community alternatives to institutional care. Specifically, the legislation required each state mental health authority to produce a plan to eliminate inappropriate institutionalization, improve the quality of care for those who need institutional care, and provide assistance to public and private agencies to facilitate screening by community mental health centers of individuals being considered for admission to a state hospital and to improve follow-up care by community mental health centers of clients discharged from mental hospitals.

It must be recognized that fundamental differences exist between P.L. 94-63, the Special Health Revenue Sharing Act, and P.L. 93-641, the National Health Planning and Resources Development Act. Mental health programs are the special concern of P.L. 94-63, while P.L. 93-641 is intended to be a comprehensive health planning mechanism. Subsequent amendments to both laws have given mental health planning more visibility as a component of health planning.

The private sector has made contributions to mental health planning through the work of advocacy groups and voluntary organizations. At the local level, community planning councils have developed special mental health plans to enable citizen decisionmaking committees to establish priorities for either developing or expanding such services as emergency psychiatric care, alcoholism programs, and children's residential treatment facilities. Mental health associations, through a network of lay and professional members, have provided leadership in proposing progressive legislative programs to improve both community and state institutional services. Private foundations have awarded grants to private and public organizations to finance mental health planning activities at local and state levels.

While private sector planning efforts have a long history, a review of the evolution of mental health planning in the United States conveys clearly the impact that federal legislation has had in shaping the structure of planning at the state and the local level. Many mental health planners agree that there is a need for a single planning system to include all health services. Until unified planning occurs, health planning agencies and mental health planning organizations will have to rely on coordination and cooperation to promote truly comprehensive health planning.

The Mental Health Planning Process

The Task Panel on Planning and Review of the President's Commission on Mental Health (1978) recommended that mental health and health planning activities be consolidated. Current requirements for state mental health planning have resulted in a top-down process. Members of the panel advocated a bottom-up approach to mental health planning because it would give a more prominent planning role to local mental health service providers and consumers. This approach also would facilitate the work of the mental health advisory committee of the local health systems agency (HSA). Furthermore, it would serve to foster a meaningful coordinated relationship between health and mental health planning.

Social workers in the mental health planning field will have to relate to state level centralized planning practices, as well as to planning that is carried out at the community or the regional level in the health systems agency. It is important for the practitioner to understand the mandated responsibilities of planning personnel at both levels. Social workers, with their community organization skills and interactional abilities, can make a significant contribution to bringing the two planning approaches into better focus by working to promote coordination between them. In the long run, improved coordination between centralized and regional planning should enhance services for clients.

The Nature of Planning

Planning is concerned with the future. Organizations must plan in order to keep a growing edge to their programs. Planning offers a vehicle for agency administrators to assess future needs, possible resources, and the variety of options that are available to the organization in meeting changing conditions.

Decisions made today by planning groups may affect service delivery for years. For example, the decision to include a day treatment center as part of a range of mental health services may affect admission and discharge patterns of a psychiatric hospital: patients who might have been hospitalized might be appropriately treated in a well-organized day program, and hospital inpatients might be discharged sooner if a day program is available to provide rehabilitation services.

Planning also implies setting goals and developing strategies and policies to attain them. It means developing a framework that will permit the organization to review current programs and propose appropriate new directions to meet short- and long-term challenges. The essential issue for planners is what should be done now to anticipate future demands on the service system.

Most planning theorists describe at least two approaches to planning. One model is rational planning, which is based upon the collection of data and their objective analysis. Hagedorn (1977) described the rational model as a process that expects its findings to be accepted because of the logical way in which the data are presented. Another planning approach, which represents a shift from the solely technical model, is participatory planning. This method stresses involvement of the people who may be affected by the planning process. The strategy is based on the view that planning is aimed at resolving an issue while at the same time creating acceptance for the approach. It also implies that those who participate in the planning process will develop some commitment to the goals of the planning endeavor. Littlestone (1973) described participatory planning as a community organization process that evolved as part of society's reponse to a variety of human problems.

In mental health planning, both approaches are needed at some stage of the planning process. Sound planning requires objective data and careful analysis. Yet, if the goal of planning is to influence future decisions, then involvement of a network of organizations and individuals is necessary.

A critical factor in planning is leadership commitment to the planning enterprise. When the agency administrator assigns a high priority to planning, other personnel will respond accordingly. If the administrator consults with his planning staff, assumes responsibility for implementing planning strategies, and communicates to department heads that he expects their cooperation with the planning proposals that he has endorsed, then the milieu for planning in the organization will be positive.

Despite the importance of planning within the context of state and federal legislation, there still remain pockets of resistance to planning. Passive resistance to making creative use of the planning staff usually surfaces when planning staff are not included in high-level administrative staff meetings or are used for routine tasks such as reviewing legislation and drafting preliminary procedures for policies that have been promulgated.

Social workers are in an ideal position to provide leadership in planning activities by the very nature of their professional education. Planning approaches show a significant overlap with social work concepts. Curriculum content about communities, program administration, and coordination of services, as well as knowledge and skill in clinical practice, are all important aspects of involving people and organizations in a cooperative undertaking.

Qualifications for Mental Health Planners

State mental health administrators were in a dilemma in the 1960s, when new federal legislation for community mental health centers stressed planning. Few individuals possessed both planning experience and mental health practice experience.

In many states, mental health laws were revised in response to the state planning efforts that were generated by the grants Congress had approved in implementing the findings of the Joint Commission on Mental Illness and Health. Many of these legislative revisions required local mental health boards to submit plans in order to qualify for state grants to finance local mental health services.

Faced with federal and state planning requirements, state mental health administrations began to devote considerable time to establishing planning positions in state offices and assisting local mental health boards to recruit planners. Qualifications for these planning positions stressed experience in mental health practice. It seemed essential that a planner of mental health services have a background in direct service provision.

Early experience with establishing planning positions suggested other qualifications. In addition to possessing mental health experience, planners should be knowledgeable about administrative procedures: supervising personnel, communicating program goals, working with governing boards and citizen groups, and overseeing financial plans. A flair for community organization is another desirable qualification. The importance of this skill is underscored by the need to involve diverse population groups and to obtain communitywide representation in the planning effort. A thorough knowledge of the health and social welfare organizational network also is helpful because mental health services frequently are supplemented by a broad array of human services in the community. Community organization skills demand an appreciation of the difficulties involved in coordinating the assortment of public and private agency services that are found in most cities. The planner should have the ability to handle interorganizational differences. Fostering cooperation on behalf of the best interests of the community demands patience and tact on the part of the planner.

Other qualifications that are considered desirable for planners include the ability to communicate clearly, to lead group discussions skillfully, and to understand and contend with the politics of planning. Familiarity with automated data systems and statistical analysis usually is required in planning positions. The planner should be able to ask the appropriate questions and to use the retrieval system for planning operations. The complex federal laws that mandate health planning—as well as mental health planning—make it necessary that planners have a comprehensive knowledge of planning legislation. They also need to understand how mental health planning must be coordinated with health planning at the regional and state levels.

The planner who understands the culture and traditions of the area for which he is responsible is in a strong position to link the current planning process with past experience. Appreciation of an area's unique characteristics facilitates interorganizational cooperation and avoids time-consuming delays caused by hurt feelings or resistance to government intervention. Clearly, the effective mental health planner should have the ability to relate easily to a wide variety of people, including professionals and laymen. In addition, the planner should be able to practice comfortably across organizational boundaries and with various levels of government officials.

Burke (1979) identified seven major functional roles of the planner that emphasize the new skills required to fulfill his responsibilities. These functional roles include the planner as analyst, organizer, broker, advocate, enabler, educator, and publicist.

Citizen Participation in Nongovernmental Statewide Planning

The work of the President's Commission on Mental Health stimulated citizen groups to play a more active role in the planning process. These advocacy groups are beginning to monitor more closely planning at both the state and the regional health systems agency level.

A nongovernmental statewide mental health planning effort was launched in Texas soon after the President's Commission on Mental Health released its study. Challenged by the commission's report, a citizens' organization was formed. Citizens for Human Development represented the state mental health association, the state association for retarded citizens, and the state organization for community mental health and mental retardation centers. The movement's stated goals were to assess the effectiveness of the state mental health and mental retardation delivery systems in meeting the needs of the people, to make recommendations for improving the service delivery systems, and to encourage local study groups to identify their communities' mental health priorities and submit recommendations to the regional health systems agencies for inclusion in the comprehensive regional health plans.

The leaders of Citizens for Human Development enlisted a broad spectrum of individuals and organizations across the state to establish a wide base of support for encouraging changes in the mental health service delivery system. The planning strategy combined a rational approach with a participatory model. Study groups in each of the twelve health regions assisted the small planning staff in the central office of Citizens for Human Development by encouraging the cooperation of local people and organizations in a statewide needs assessment. The concentrated efforts of many volunteers throughout the state produced the first statewide mental health and mental retardation needs assessment ever attempted in Texas (Citizens for Human Development, 1981).

The results of the survey of needs were tabulated on both a statewide and a regional (health systems agency) basis. Local study groups utilized the needs assessment data for their regions, advising their mental health and mental retardation center boards about findings and the implications for priorities. Personnel of health systems agencies were urged to include survey findings in regional health plans. At the state level, representatives of Citizens for Human Development shared survey results with the state mental health authority and gave testimony before legislative committees concerned with appropriations for the state mental health and mental retardation programs.

Nongovernmental statewide planning efforts can be effective only if there are strong linkages between the central planning office of the organization and citizen study committees in outlying regions. Local volunteer study groups need ongoing support and direction from the central office. It also helps for them to be aware of the progress of other citizen study groups throughout the state. The central office can facilitate the sharing of information through a regular newsletter or some similar communication vehicle.

Grass-roots participation in statewide planning puts to the test the concept that people will take an interest in the planning of public services. Maintaining citizen interest presents a sterling challenge in participatory planning. However, rarely do advocacy groups achieve all their goals on the first attempt. The complex task of meeting the changing needs of the mentally ill or those with relatively minor health problems appears to be a never ending struggle. The unmet needs that the citizens' planning organization in Texas identified have given these volunteers an incentive to maintain their advocacy efforts. Perhaps the unresolved issues in developing realistic, comprehensive services will be sufficient to sustain the planning efforts of other nongovernmental groups.

Governmental Planning at the State Level

A recurring criticism of state mental health planning is that the effort is often an annual activity that reflects the constraints of ongoing programs. It is not uncommon for state level planners in governmental agencies to take a plan from the previous year and update it. However, changes in federal legislation often furnish an incentive to develop a new plan that involves a significant number of people throughout the mental health system in a dynamic planning endeavor.

Setting Goals and Objectives
Based on Preliminary Assessments

In building a new state plan, the first task of the planning office is to make certain that changes in policy or the impact of new laws are accommodated in the annual plan. A careful review of the existing plan may show the necessity of plan revision because of budget changes or new interagency working relationships. Revised standards of accrediting committees, affecting patient care criteria, also must be considered.

Policy changes often reflect new patterns of service delivery. For example, mental hospitals in some states have a system of outreach clinics to serve discharged patients, especially those patients living in rural areas. As community mental health centers have grown in number and expanded into regional service areas with a comprehensive array of services, there is the possibility of an overlap of services, with duplication of effort. At some point, the state mental health authority will take cognizance of this development and promulgate a new policy that community mental health centers are responsible for follow-up care of discharged patients. This policy change must be reflected in the new state plan, with appropriate modifications in the budgets of hospitals and additional financial allocations made to the mental health centers taking over follow-up services.

The implications of changes in the mental health system should be reviewed in the goal setting section of the plan. Subtle changes in the patient population will affect the future allocations of funds and thus influence planning considerations. The following issues are relevant in this context:

Are hospitals becoming filled with chronically ill patients?

Are admissions reflecting an increasing number of young people?

What has been the trend in allocating resources between mental retardation facilities and mental hospitals?

What has been the trend in allocating resources between mental hospitals and community services?

What role does the hospice play in the mental health delivery system?

In what ways is the mental health delivery system serving patients with physical disabilities and terminally ill patients?

What classes of employees are experiencing unusually high turnover rates?

The planning process may identify areas in which policies are vague and unclear, so it is important that the planning staff annually review all policies and laws that affect the operation of the mental health system. Review of policies as part of the planning process will offer opportunities for policy revisions where indicated. Working with department heads will enable the planning staff to identify new areas of agreement and to participate in the discussions that generate new goals and objectives for the organization. These goals and objectives should be ideals toward which the state mental health program strives. The goals of advocacy groups such as the state mental health association and the state association for retarded citizens should be included in the goal setting. In view of the investment of time and effort by members of the President's Commission on Mental Health, it would be appropriate also to include the challenging goals of the commission.

Needs Assessment

Mental health planners usually define needs assessment as a research and planning activity with the objective of identifying a community's mental health service needs. A vital part of needs assessment is to seek information from several sources: the agency that presently provides the service and the population or geographic area served by the mental health agency. The needs assessment program attempts to collect data that will assist the mental health planners to determine the scope and type of mental health needs in the community, evaluate the effectiveness of the current service delivery system, and design new programs and services in response to unmet needs.

Planning staff should be cautious in relying on staff perceptions of community need instead of eliciting the information from consumers or those close to consumers of services. Another problem that arises in assessing utilization of services is that the data reflect actual use and do not take into account those individuals who could have used the service but for some reason did not.

The National Institute of Mental Health has published a helpful manual for mental health planning personnel (Warheit, Bell, and Schwab, 1977). Five needs assessment approaches are offered, along with materials that the planner can adapt to meet specific study requirements. The manual has a practical orientation and should be of assistance to those doing community studies.

State level planners usually have a rich data bank that gives them information about the volume of services provided in any area during any given time period. They have a ready network for gathering community need information through the data collection resources of community mental health centers in the state. Social workers practicing in centers can gain experience with needs assessment by participating in this phase of the planning process. Social workers also can make a contribution to the comprehensiveness of the data gathering operation by giving special attention to identifying mental health problems among low-income groups, minorities, the elderly, and other disadvantaged or high-risk groups.

Inventories of Resources

A third component in developing a state mental health plan involves producing an inventory of resources that satisfies federal requirements and meets the needs of the state mental health authority.

Directories of resources frequently are out of date by the time information is collected, organized, and published. However, inventories do provide a baseline of readily accessible information and they furnish a reasonable guideline for setting priorities in each geographic region or catchment area. Inventories may include the following resources:

1. planning programs in the state that deal with mental health services, facilities, and manpower (identifying data—e.g., names and addresses of organizations—along with descriptions of responsibilities, should be included)
2. provider organizations, including professional societies, with their membership lists and the geographic locations of members
3. mental health facilities, including hospitals with psychiatric facilities, mental health centers, nursing homes, child guidance clinics, private residential resources, and outpatient services
4. other public agencies, such as councils of governments, health systems agencies, city and county health departments, and public universities, including psychiatry departments of medical schools, schools of nursing, schools of social work, and other training centers for mental health manpower
5. mental health and mental health related advocacy groups, such as the state mental health association and its affiliates, the state society for autistic citizens, and other associations for handicapped individuals

Resource inventories should be organized, as much as possible, to enable the planning office to make some determination about the adequacy of services directed at meeting the mental health needs of the target population. For example, the number of psychiatric beds in the community should be related to the number of people living in the area.

Establishing Short- and Long-range Objectives

The setting of goals and objectives is a key element in the planning process. Objectives usually are regarded as measurable stages on the way to achieving a goal. In mental health planning, objectives should relate to prevention, care and treatment, rehabilitation, resource development, manpower needs, and linkages between state hospital facilities and community mental health centers. The objectives should be based upon an estimate of the magnitude of the problems that are anticipated and the extent to which projected resources may be used toward meeting these problems.

The state mental health planning staff have a responsibility to communicate to others their tentative goals and objectives and encourage reactions to their proposals. Not only should other mental health staff of the agency be involved in the process, but also other participants should comment in order to build a network of support for the planning effort. Others who might participate in the setting of objectives are advocacy groups, board members of community mental health centers, staff from mental hospitals, key members of legislative committees, representatives from the executive branch, and staff from both the state health department planning office and the various regional health systems agencies.

Ultimately, priorities have to be identified, and frequently disputes arise in the process. The planner's role is to promote consensus and maintain open communication among the disagreeing parties. Since the legislature usually makes the final decision about priorities, the planning office should try to get adequate details to the appropriate committees of the legislative body to assist them with their decision.

Implementation Schedule

Once a plan has been developed and priorities selected, the mental health planner has the responsibility for preparing a report that outlines the accomplishments of the planning process and distributing the report to all interested individuals and organizations. There should be adequate time for review of the planning results. Comments should be encouraged and time scheduled for the comments to be considered and included in the final plan. A schedule for implementation of the plan should include recommended legislation, financing expectations, identification of public and private organizations that might assume responsibility for the development of programs, and procedures for evaluating progress. Some provision for updating the state plan should be included in the implementation schedule.

It should be noted that the planning process does not flow in an orderly, step-by-step manner. Some phases of the planning process may be delayed while specific data are being collected and analyzed. Study committees may not meet scheduled deadlines. The collection of information for the inventory of existing programs and resources may continue throughout the various stages of the planning process. The planning staff may have to interrupt their schedule to prepare periodic reports for members of the administrative staff who carry responsibility for appearing before legislative groups or other public organizations.

Social workers can make significant contributions throughout the planning process because of their ability to work with diverse groups and their knowledge of the network of human services. Field work assignments in state mental health planning offices offer social work students a rich variety of learning experiences that complement content taught in the classroom. The three-year Community Mental Health Curriculum Project of the Council on Social Work Education noted that innovative field assignments often constituted the only component that could be identified clearly with the community mental health curriculum (Rubin, 1979).

Community Mental Health Planning

President Kennedy's call for a bold, new approach to solving the nation's mounting mental health problems launched the community mental health center movement in 1963. The new approach to the care of the mentally ill implied a departure from previous efforts and offered a new conceptual framework for the provision of mental health services.

Several features distinguish community mental health programs. First, federal legislation makes each community mental health center responsible for a particular catchment area. Second, the community mental health orientation emphasizes the provision and coordination of comprehensive services. Continuity of care for individuals in the community mental health center's treatment program is a concept that is receiving increasing attention as stronger linkages are developed between community and institutional programs.

An innovative characteristic of the community approach is the emphasis on a rational planning process to identify unmet community needs. Mental health planners in the community review existing patterns of service utilization, identify populations within the community that are considered to be at high risk for developing mental illness, and recommend priorities for the future delivery of services. Planners are giving increasing attention to preventive strategies and are seeking ways to reduce sources of stress in the community (Wittman and Arch, 1980).

Citizen participation is another distinguishing characteristic of community mental health programs. Citizen involvement grew out of the belief that the mental health professional should not be the only authority on the mental health needs of the community. Instead, the staff of the mental health center should involve citizen advisory groups in identifying local needs and in proposing programs to meet future community service needs. The concept of community participation in the affairs of the mental health program underscores the meaning of the term "community" in community mental health.

Citizen participation in community mental health program planning involves former and potential consumers of the center's services, as well as advocates for improving community programs. Advisory committees include individuals who live in the center's catchment area. Citizens are encouraged to become involved in the review of programs, to identify for staff the unserved or underserved sectors of the catchment area, and to participate in decisionmaking affecting the center's development. Dynamic participation by representatives of the community has the potential of increasing the responsiveness and accountability of service providers and enhancing the possibility that potential consumers and the general public will become more aware of the availability and accessibility of services (Miller, 1979).

Unfortunately, citizen participation in the decisionmaking process of community mental health centers often has been accompanied by conflict and bitter controversy. It is essential that specific tasks of citizen committees be clearly understood by both the staff of the center and community groups. Frequently, the citizen volunteer develops a strong loyalty to a particular service or neighborhood facility. Other citizen volunteers may develop similar commitments in other areas of a center's broad program. Such personal commitments tend to fragment the operations of the total center and create dilemmas for the governing board in establishing priorities for the general welfare of the total community. Another factor in the conflict that sometimes arises among the participating citizen groups is the unrealistic expectations staff and citizens have of each other. Unfulfilled expectations can lead to disappointment, anger, and frustration (Salber, 1970).

While many problems do surface when there is representative community involvement in the community mental health administration and planning process, citizen participation still represents an excellent method for eliciting support for the program. More attention needs to be given to finding creative ways to use citizens' energy and enthusiasm in enriching local programs (Morrison, Holdridge-Crane, and Smith, 1978).

Social workers long have recognized the therapeutic gains of participation. Because of the profession's belief in the merits of the democratic process, social work has a considerable stake in the development of citizen participation in community mental health programs in particular and in the human services generally.

The planning of local services should capitalize on the interests of citizens to monitor the services that are being delivered. The planning enterprise also should appeal to consumers and advocates because changing conditions in society accelerate the need for either new services or new ways to deliver services. Any local planning effort, then, should include a participatory approach to augment the ongoing rational planning process of the professional staff of the center.

Local Planning Strategies

In community mental health, planning at the local level initiates the process that the Task Panel on Planning and Review of the President's Commission on Mental Health (1978) called a bottom-up approach. This means that planning recommendations ideally should begin at the local level and move through several stages until the recommendations are incorporated into the official state plan. The panel also stressed the importance of coordinating local mental health planning activities with the planning process of the mental health advisory committee of the regional health systems agency. By working together, the two local planning endeavors can supplement each other and produce a realistic regional mental health plan that will become part of the region's comprehensive health plan.

Planning in the local community mental health program can utilize several approaches, but consideration should be given to applying basic health planning methods wherever appropriate. The elements of planning are more or less the same regardless of the field of study. The components include identifying the problem, setting objectives, assessing resources, analyzing possible solutions, developing a plan of action, implementing recommendations, and evaluating results. Planning related to health requires the efforts of both consumers and providers of services under current health planning guidelines. There have been some weaknesses in the use of consumer or citizen participation in the planning process because planning bodies have presumed that the citizen participant represented, if not all the consumer population, at least most consumers. There also has been a tendency toward professional domination of decisions and ineffective blending of consumer thinking into the planning process (Flexner and Berkowitz, 1979). The risk in underestimating the contributions of citizen volunteers is that the staff may fail to develop programs that are sensitive and responsive to the needs of the community.

Identifying Local Mental Health Problems

Various techniques may be used to assist the staff and citizen volunteers to gather data that will identify major problem areas. Three means are personal interviews, telephone interviews, and mailed questionnaires. Personal interviews are more costly than either telephone surveys or mailed questionnaires, but this method permits a more comprehensive coverage of the questions.

Care must be taken in constructing the instrument that is to be used in gathering the data for identifying problems. There is a vast literature available to those who have the responsibility for developing such instruments (Warheit, Bell, and Schwab, 1977). The survey should address the areas of concern that will help to determine the current mental health needs of the community and to identify populations that are either unserved or poorly served. The questionnaire must be constructed in a way that facilitates organization and tabulation of collected data.

Most mental health centers set their ultimate goals in broad terms, such as improving the mental health of the community or reducing dramatically the number of patients who are admitted to state hospitals. Ultimate goals may be stated as both long- and short-term objectives.

Proposing Behavioral Objectives
to Meet Identified Problems

The staff and planning committee may decide to increase the time spent on follow-up care of patients returning to the community from state hospitals in order to prevent rehospitalization and may make that goal an objective. Another objective might be to set up a screening program for preschool children to insure early detection of emotional problems.

Assessing Resources

The inventory of local resources may list all agencies related to mental health and their manpower capabilities. Often the private sector is overlooked in a survey of resources, but privately practicing professional people carry a significant amount of the mental health caseload of a community. Counseling resources in the public schools also may be neglected. The community planning councils in most communities usually are familiar with resources that are being developed but may not be operational at the time resources are assessed.

Generating Possible Program Solutions

After analyzing the identified needs and the available resources, the staff and the citizen advisory group must develop appropriate program objectives.

Mental health center personnel have been hard pressed for the most part in meeting basic demands for service. This activity has left staff with little energy to devote to developing innovative programs to meet new needs. A number of centers in Texas, for example, have experienced reductions in services because state and local public tax funds are insufficient to replace expiring federal grant programs. However, it is important for staff and citizen advisory groups to monitor community responses to the lack of comprehensive services to meet special needs. The rising rate of suicide among teenagers is a concern to parents and community leaders. The increasing evidence of child abuse among young families also demands some program consideration from mental health personnel.

The relationship of certain problems to the lack of services needs to be communicated to the community through citizen advisory groups and advocacy organizations. Education programs aimed at helping parents better to understand the developmental needs of their children would be one possible way to reduce child abuse. Target groups would be newly married couples or couples having their first child. Seminars in junior and senior high schools to acquaint youth with crisis center services and telephone hotline emergency services could be developed to reduce the incidence of suicide among young people.

Developing a Plan of Action

Exploration of program possibilities to meet recognized needs is important, but this is wasted effort if the discussions are not translated into a plan to achieve stated objectives. For example, a plan for combating teenage suicide might involve the recruitment of interested parties from parent groups in the schools and from youth organizations. Similarly, a program to reduce the incidence of child abuse might solicit support from the medical society, law enforcement officials, and child welfare staff.

Implementing Planning Recommendations

Support may be garnered for implementing planning recommendations if concerned citizens, who have been identified in the action plan, are mobilized to create public response to the need. Educational materials may be developed for distribution to the public. Civic leaders may be interviewed on radio or local television. Presentations before civic clubs and professional groups could present study findings and recommendations.

Social work staff have an investment in implementing planning recommendations to meet human needs. Social workers frequently are the ones who discover the need and have the responsibility for doing something about the problem. Any program that can prevent a tragedy, by providing much needed services, will enable social workers to spend more time on other preventive activities and on reducing stressful conditions among the people of the community.

Evaluating Results

Campaigns to mobilize community support for preventive and other programs will have to be evaluated. What has been the response to the educational materials that were distributed? Are community leaders ready to provide financial support for proposed programs? Has the mere public discussion of the problem areas resulted in any gains (e.g., reduction in teenage suicide and child abuse)?

Newly recommended programs do not get implemented for a variety of reasons. However, the merits of the planning process, which brings certain needs to the community's attention, should not be underestimated. The process may have more value than planning staff can document. In the long run, the community mental health center is meeting its responsibility by publicizing locally those areas of urgent need.

Trends and Issues

The Task Panel on Planning and Review of the President's Commission on Mental Health (1978) issued a warning to social workers who currently are in mental health planning positions or who contemplate practicing in planning offices. The panel reported that state level planning in the human services is becoming so complex that planning is in danger of becoming bureaucratized. Under these circumstances, mental health participation in cooperative planning endeavors is very limited.

At the community level, problems of territory have arisen. Communication obstacles are more frequent than examples of cooperation among agency representatives. Social work, with its long history of encouraging collaboration among human services agencies on behalf of the recipients of services, can provide community leadership in removing barriers to cooperative planning. Responsible planning implies close coordination among service providers and between levels of government.

Because of differences in federal planning laws, mental health planning is in an unusual position. Many mental health programs established under P.L. 94-63 must be implemented under the provisions of P.L. 93-641, the National Health Planning and Resources Development Act. The certificate of need program has special implications for mental health program planning. The addition of a new mental health service must be reviewed in the planning process to determine whether or not a certificate of need is required. A certificate of need is required if the new service results in any capital expenditure or involves annual operating costs of at least $75,000. Federal grants to support mental health services in the community must be approved by the health planning authorities whenever the grant involves new or expanded services that are covered by the certificate of need program. Social work planners must be alert to the dichotomies in federal legislation and provide organizational safeguards to assure continuity of services to consumers. It is hoped that the conflicts in the two federal laws soon will be resolved and that a comprehensive, unitary planning process will replace the current dual planning system. However, the direction of the Reagan administration regarding social legislation suggests that planning requirements will be drastically reduced, if not eliminated, in some areas.

The issue of citizen participation in mental health planning and decisionmaking merits more attention from social work researchers. Despite commitment to the concept of citizen participation in facilitating change, there has not been warm acceptance of citizen groups in mental health planning by social workers or other mental health professionals. Citizen participants have received only limited acceptance—often with overt reservations (Miller, 1979).

Social work education has not distinguished itself in the development of new knowledge relevant to citizen participation. Because of the failure of mental health professionals to accept with enthusiasm the efforts of citizens in program planning and decisionmaking, social workers should be trained as students to deal with the attitudes of their professional colleagues. Possible ameliorative actions include more careful selection of citizen participants and training workshops to increase their competence.

Students also should be prepared to work with citizen groups. They should receive instruction in the contribution of grass-roots movements to welfare reform and to upgrading mental health services for more than a century. Social work classes should study methods that may be used to involve citizens as members of policymaking boards and citizen advisory committees and as advocates for special programs. In field work, students should have the opportunity to work with a citizen group that is involved in community decisionmaking. Students also should be given an opportunity to develop a framework to assess the quality of citizen participation in mental health planning activities.

While the contributions of volunteers frequently are acknowledged, usually their activities center on areas that have been designated by professional staff members. In view of the increasing role volunteers will play in mental health planning activities under federal law, it seems appropriate that social work should document the contributions of citizen participants to the mental health agency and the greater community.

Finally, social work practitioners should look critically at the mental health planning process at both the state and the local level. Because planning is required by federal and state legislation, there is a real possibility that the process will emphasize increasingly the structure of planning and neglect the human dimensions that are the goals of the enterprise. Social workers in mental health planning roles also should become advocates for the plans they help to formulate; planning is an empty exercise if implementation is not forthcoming.

REFERENCES

BACHRACH, L. L. "Planning Mental Health Services for Chronic Patients." *Hospital and Community Psychiatry* 1979, *30*(6):387–393.

BEECH, R. P., FIESTER, A. R., and SILVERMAN, W. H. "Demographic Data and Mental Health Planning." *Administration in Mental Health* 1976, *3*(Spring):166–173.

BLOOM, B. L. *Community Mental Health: A Historical and Critical Analysis.* Morristown, N.J.: General Learning, 1973.

BURKE, E. M. *A Participatory Approach to Urban Planning.* New York: Human Sciences, 1979.

CAMPBELL, L. A. "Consumer Participation in Planning Social Service Programs." *Social Work* 1979, *24*(2):159–162.

Citizens for Human Development. *Report on a Statewide Citizen Approach to Assessing Mental Health and Mental Retardation Needs in Texas.* Austin: Citizens for Human Development, 1981.

DEMONE, H. W., JR., and HARSHBARGER, D. *The Planning and Administration of Human Services.* New York: Behavioral Publications, 1973.

Federal Register, March 26, 1980, pp. 20, 026–20, 044.

FLEXNER, W. A., and BERKOWITZ, E. N. "Marketing Research in Health Services Planning: A Model." *Public Health Reports* 1979, *94*(6):503–513.

HAGEDORN, H. *A Manual on State Mental Health Planning.* Rockville, Md.: National Institute of Mental Health, 1977.

Joint Commission on Mental Illness and Health. *Action for Mental Health.* New York: Basic Books, 1961.

KANE, T. "Citizen Participation in Decision Making: Myth or Strategy." *Administration in Mental Health* 1975, *4*(Summer):29–34.

LAMSON, W. C. "The Role of the Psychiatric Social Worker in Mental Health Programs—in a National Program." *Journal of Psychiatric Social Work* 1954, *23*(3):142–147.

LITTLESTONE, R. "Planning in Mental Health." In S. Feldman (ed.), *The Administration of Mental Health Services.* Springfield, Ill.: Thomas, 1973.

MILLER, S. O. "Citizen Participation in Community Mental Health Programs." In A. J. Katz (ed.), *Community Mental Health: Issues for Social Work Practice and Education.* New York: Council on Social Work Education, 1979.

MORRISON, J. K., HOLDRIDGE-CRANE, S., and SMITH, J. E. "Citizen Participation in Community Mental Health." *Community Mental Health Review* 1978, *3*(3):1–9.

RUBIN, A. *Community Mental Health in the Social Work Curriculum.* New York: Council on Social Work Education, 1979.

SALBER, E. J. "Community Participation in Neighborhood Health Centers." *New England Journal of Medicine* 1970, *283*(10):515–518.

SCHULBERG, H. C., BOARD, G., III, and SHAEFFER, D. N. "The Balanced Service System and the Planning of Community Mental Health Programs." *Administration in Mental Health* 1979, *7*(Winter):95–111.

SPIEGEL, A. D., and HYMAN, H. H. *Basic Health Planning Methods.* Germantown, Md.: Aspen, 1978.

Task Panel on Planning and Review, President's Commission on Mental Health. *Task Panel Reports Submitted to the President's Commission on Mental Health,* vol. 2. Washington, D.C.: U.S. Government Printing Office, 1978.

U.S. Congress, House Committee on Interstate and Foreign Commerce. *Hearings on H.R. 2550, National Neuropsychiatric Institute Act.* 79th Cong., 1st sess., 1945, p. 36.

U.S. Congress, Senate Committee on Appropriations. *Hearings, Departments of Labor and Health, Education, and Welfare Appropriations for 1963,* pt. II. 87th Cong., 2d sess., 1962, p. 1585.

WARHEIT, G. J., BELL, R. A., and SCHWAB, J. J. *Needs Assessment Approaches: Concepts and Methods.* Rockville, Md.: National Institute of Mental Health, 1977.

WERNERT, T. M. "Planning for Mental Health Services." *Administration in Mental Health* 1979, *6*(Spring):216–234

WITTMAN, F. D., and ARCH, M. "Task Force Report: Sociophysical Settings and Mental Health: Opportunities for Mental Health Service Planning." *Community Mental Health Journal* 1980, *16*(1):45–61.

CHAPTER 8

Community Organization

Mark Tarail

THIS CHAPTER describes briefly the rise of community organization in social work and in mental health. I also discuss some of the principles and concepts underpinning the use of community organization in mental health and examine mental health and related programs utilizing community organization. The chapter closes with a review of current trends in mental health service delivery that relate to community organization.

Community Organization in Social Work

Since the development and proliferation of graduate schools of social work in the late 1920s and 1930s in this country, many schools of social work have provided preparation in community organization. In some schools, students have been able to elect community organization as a track in graduate training; in other schools, all students have been exposed to generic courses in community organization (Brager and Specht, 1973). In the past few years some schools have developed a track in administration and policy and provided community organization education in connection with the training program in administration.

In the 1930s, 1940s, and 1950s, jobs for community organizers as such were available in the various fields of social work. Social workers trained in community organization were hired for these positions. In the past few years social workers have been employed in diverse positions involving community organization in health, mental health, and social service agencies but without the title "community organizer." (See, for example, Rothman, 1979, for a discussion of models of community organization practice.) Social workers with community organization skills are in jobs as health and social services planners; as administrators in human service agencies, including health and mental health facilities; and as liaison workers and co-ordinators in various human services.

Community organization technology and workers trained in this area, then, have proven useful in planning, administration, and interagency liaison. The field of community development also relies heavily on community organization. This field has been expanding since the 1950s, with the proliferation of so-called community antipoverty programs, the increased need for planning and organization in large housing projects, and the relatively recent establishment of local community development agencies by cities and counties in both urban and rural areas (Ferguson, 1963). The rise of the community mental health movement in the late 1950s and early 1960s stimulated the use of community organization technology and the employment of community organizers for the first time in the mental health field.

Community Organization in Mental Health

Community organization, with its unique ideology and technology, increasingly was used in psychiatric and mental health agencies and facilities in the middle 1960s in the United States as a consequence of the rise of the community mental health movement and the establishment of comprehensive community mental health centers throughout the country. During World War II, with the identification of psychiatric problems in large numbers of recruits drafted for the Armed Services, and the postwar years, a new national awareness developed concerning mental illness. Accordingly, a number of epidemiological studies on the incidence and prevalence of mental illness in the general population were conducted (e.g., Srole, Langner, Michael, Opler, and Rennie, 1962). These studies provided evidence of the high incidence and prevalence rates of mental illness in all groups in the general population. They also pointed to the lack of mental health services for large sections of the population and identified a statistically significant relationship between pathogenic social factors, such as poverty, unemployment, and racism, and the incidence and severity of mental illness.

The Joint Commission on Mental Illness and Health (1961) confirmed the findings of the epidemiological studies done in the 1950s. The commission also noted that few mental health services were available for large sections of the population in the United States and that available services often were not accessible to the population that needed them. The lack of accessibility often reflected the policy of mental health agencies not to accept for treatment individuals who were not covered by third-party reimbursements or could not afford to pay fees. The location of the facility and the agency's intake criteria, based on diagnostic category, severity of illness, or age, also discouraged utilization of available services. The commission recommended that a national program be established involving the development of a network of comprehensive community mental health centers. Through such centers, mental health services, including preventive programs, would be made available and accessible to all sections of the population. These new facilities would be located in catchment areas containing 100,000–200,000 people and would be funded by the federal government, with matching support from state, local, county, and city governments.

In 1963 the Kennedy administration introduced and Congress passed the Community Mental Health Centers Act to implement the program. For the first time in the history of health services, a national social policy recognized that the health and illness of all the people of the United States were the responsibility of the federal government and that federal funds should be made available for the planning, operation, and staffing of mental health facilities. Through the Community Mental Health Centers Act of 1963 and its amendments the federal funds were used as seed money; that is, the funds were provided in decreasing amounts over an eight-year period with the idea that local, county, city, and state governments would be able to pick up the full cost of the centers at the end of eight years. The federal government also defined the mandates, objectives, and the required elements of service for these comprehensive community mental health centers and tied these mandates to the obtaining of federal funds and to a process of monitoring the services of the federally funded facilities.

By 1975, ten years later, close to a thousand community mental health centers were in operation across the country (National Institute of Mental Health, 1979). In 1980, approximately eight-hundred such centers existed in the United States. In addition, many psychiatric facilities and freestanding family and child guidance agencies and clinics began to change the nature of their services. Many states also became interested in creating an integrated system of mental health services; community mental health ideology and practice began to proliferate.

The mandates of the community mental health centers and the new tasks taken on by other mental health agencies and facilities during this period required the implementation of new goals and programs. In addition to providing diagnostic and treatment services, mental health centers now had to offer preventive and community mental health education programs in and with local populations, consultation and education services to other agencies and institutions in local communities, and rehabilitation and restoration services. The federally funded designated centers also were required to make their services accessible twenty-four hours a day, seven days a week, for regular as well as emergency and crisis intervention purposes; to develop outreach mental health programs for neighborhoods and high-risk populations; and, for the first time in the history of health services in this country, to provide services to all individuals residing in a given service, or catchment, area regardless of ability to pay, age, sex, nationality, ethnicity, religion, diagnostic category, or severity of illness. Mandated also was a new emphasis on the participation of community leaders, representing patients and clients, in decisionmaking through community advisory boards and community governing boards, with defined powers in the areas of policy, budgeting, and the hiring of leadership personnel. In addition, a planning process involving other agencies in the local community and community leaders had to be utilized as a basis for the establishment of a community mental health center.

It was precisely in the new community mental health centers and in the early stages of the community mental health movement that the psychiatrists, psychologists, social workers, and nurses who had been providing traditional mental health services found that they did not have the skills and the ability to implement many of the requirements and processes involved in planning, in community organization, and in the provision of services in the areas of prevention, consultation, and education. Community organization was found to be a ready-made methodology and technology appropriate to this new system of mental health services, and social workers trained in community organization were employed in these new mental health settings to help implement a variety of programs.

Principles and Concepts of Community Organization in Mental Health

Underpinning the special skills and technologies identified with community organization are a number of principles and concepts unique to the practice of community organization in community mental health programs. These concepts have been identified over the past fifteen years as community organization has been applied in mental health settings.

Knowledge of Mental Health

Community organizers operating in a mental health setting must be knowledgeable about mental health, psychiatry, and clinical services. While some of the techniques of community organization are useful in all settings, their successful application in the field of mental health requires familiarity with mental health problems and the types of therapeutic intervention utilized by the agency.

Task versus Process

A long-standing conflict exists in community organization between those who believe that their objective is the process of organization itself and those who feel that community organization should be task oriented. In the field of mental health, experience has demonstrated that community organization appears to be most effective when it is task and goal oriented and that the process is a means of achieving the task or the goal. Actually, the process and the goal can be conceived as integrated since effective goals require effective means and processes can be effective only in relation to essential and effective objectives (Brager and Specht, 1973).

Change and Action Orientation

It is generally accepted that the clinical treatment process in mental health is oriented toward changing intrapsychic mechanisms in the personality system of the patient or client and toward re-forming the ways in which the patient functions in the various components of daily life. Community organization technology in mental health is aimed at creating change in the attitudes and perceptions of consumers of services, community leaders, and providers of other human services concerning mental health and mental illness, the mental health agency, and the need for and utilization of mental health services. Community organization also has been helpful in creating institutional change as mental health agencies have evolved from traditional intramural psychiatric facilities into contemporary community service agencies and have abandoned preoccupation with inpatient care in favor of an emphasis on ambulatory and outreach services.

Thus, community organization tends to be most effective when it is action oriented. For instance, a fact-finding study to identify community leaders preparatory to the establishment of a community board is aimed at the creation of a representative and effective community board. A study of mental health needs in a local population is aimed at influencing the priorities and policies of the service programs (Dodson, 1966).

Building Connections

One of the primary contributions of community organization in mental health is to help the mental health facility build appropriate and effective interagency referral and service coordination with agencies providing other services required by mental patients, including health facilities, schools, and social services. Most patients and clients seeking the psychiatric treatment and the mental health interventions provided by the mental health agency also need concrete social, health, and educational services in order to be able to function with some degree of effectiveness. The human services system is fragmented into various bureaucratic, independent agencies that are difficult for patients and clients to negotiate on their own.

The community organizer, acting on behalf of the mental health facility, can establish formal as well as informal interagency connections in order to coordinate human services around the needs of individuals and families with mental health problems (Perlman and Gurin, 1972). Community organizers have done this through establishing local neighborhood or county service agency councils. They also have developed interagency referral mechanisms, interagency committees, and quid pro quo relationships wherein the mental health facility provides in-service training, consultation, and immediate help to the staff and clients of other agencies in return for expeditious service to its patients and clients by these facilities.

Integration of Fact-finding with Action

Fact-finding in community organization should be action oriented not only in relation to agency goals and policy priorities, as noted earlier, but also in the very process of fact-finding. A fundamental principle here is that whoever will implement the action to be taken as the result of the identification of the facts should participate in the planning of the fact-finding research and even in some of the fact-finding. Such involvement maximizes the results consequent upon the fact-finding.

Participation Process

Community organizers tend to be experts in the process of committee work and in the formation and activities of coalitions. In community organization, the concept is to insure the greatest participation of the widest variety of individuals in the various group meetings in the community and within the mental health agency. The principle involved is that maximum results are produced by maximum participation in the deliberations within group structures and processes. A subprinciple is that participation in the group process should be based upon an open system of peer level contributions among the members of the committee or group.

Integration of Structure and Function

An important contribution of community organization is to conceptualize and perceive a service system or a program within the agency or the community as possessing structures and functions that are integrated in practice. Structure and function cannot be separated. The structure of an operation, agency, group, or program often determines and limits the function, and the nature of the function frequently influences the character of the structure. Separating function and structure tends to diminish efficiency and effectiveness.

For example, outpatient medical clinics of general hospitals in large U.S. cities frequently offer fragmented medical services and a large number of specialty and subspecialty clinics. In many voluntary hospitals these clinics are staffed mainly by rotating residents and interns and by voluntary attending physicians, who provide one to two hours of service a week in the clinics in return for bed privileges in the inpatient units for their private patients. The clinic patient often does not see the same doctor twice during the course of treatment for an illness and frequently is treated in several specialty clinics for different conditions. The Joint Commission on Accreditation of Hospitals and the federal government recently mandated the organization of outpatient services in the form of primary care, a relatively new functional approach to the management of patients (Joint Commission on Accreditation of Hospitals, 1978). Under this plan, the patient sees the same doctor from the beginning to the end of the illness, with the primary physician coordinating all services and subspecialists needed by the patient (See Curiel, Brochstein, Cheney, and Adams, 1979). The traditional structure of fragmented outpatient subspecialty clinics prevents the primary care function from being carried out effectively. On the other hand, this new primary care function requires a new structure involving the establishment of a primary care clinic in the outpatient department (sometimes called a comprehensive medical clinic) through which all patients enter the system. In this primary clinic, a primary physician is assigned to the patient. Subspecialists are assigned to the primary clinic and become members of an interspecialty and interdisciplinary team coordinated by the primary physician, providing an organized, complex treatment plan for the patient. In this model the structure is a reflection of the function and is consonant with the purpose. In the older model, the structure is not consonant with the function and changes the function from an integrated form of medical practice to the more traditional, fragmented form of medical practice.

Manifest and Latent Power

Mental Health agencies are constantly faced with conflicts and competition for power and authority within the agency itself, in relationships with other agencies, and in the community. Examples include competition or conflict between various professional disciplines (e.g., psychiatrists versus psychologists versus social workers); among divisions and departments of the agency (e.g., inpatient versus outpatient programs); with other agencies providing mental health or related services (e.g., child mental health clinic versus public school mental disability service, or general hospital psychiatric services versus state psychiatric hospital); among ethnic, social, and economic groups in the local community; and between community leaders and consumer representatives, on the one hand, and administrators and service providers, on the other hand. Two community organization principles are involved in such disputes.

First, one must appreciate the differences between manifest, or formal, power and latent, or informal, authority. In this connection, leaders who hold formal authority and titles may not have actual power. Establishment of relationships with both formal and informal leaders is essential to the effective administration of an agency, to program implementation, and to community organization. Likewise, inherent strains and conflicts between manifest and latent power may be utilized creatively to enhance both levels of authority or to create needed institutional and social change (Health Policy Advisory Center, May and Dec. 1969, and May and June 1970).

Second, organizers working with groups competing for power and authority have found the principle of mutual advocacy to be most useful. This principle reflects a partnership between providers and consumers, between staff and administration, or between a particular mental health agency and other agencies with interfacing programs; relying on a formal agreement or common objectives, each party benefits from joint processes and activities (Tarail, 1972).

Interface between Clinical and Nonclinical Processes

An interface between clinical services and nonclinical community organization processes and programs is essential in a mental health setting. Some community mental health centers have separated community organization, prevention, consultation, and education from clinical services. This separation has tended to produce conflict and competition.

Community organization is not an end in itself in mental health. It is an instrument to enhance clinical services and to organize the channels through which preventive and outreach services can be provided to individuals and families who need them and who have been unreachable by traditional psychiatric facilities. Community organization also provides additional means to enhance the agency's ability to achieve its goals. Thus, mental health centers like the Maimonides Community Mental Health Center in Brooklyn, New York, have found it fruitful for clinicians to participate in outreach programs and for community organizers to participate in clinical services decisionmaking.

Integration of Community Organization with
Administration and Program Evaluation

Community organization often is useful in administration and program evaluation. For instance, in mental health administration community organization skills are essential to creating an effective public and community relations program; to organizing, developing, and defining the responsibilities of a community board; to fact-finding concerning mental health needs and community services to serve those needs; and to building community support and local constituencies in the interests of the agency specifically and mental health services in general (Tarail, 1979). In program evaluation, community organization technology has been found helpful in identifying the perceptions of both community residents and other agencies concerning the services of the mental health facility and in studying and assessing the service priorities and practices of the mental health agency in relation to the mental health needs of the local community.

Indigenous Roots

Since community organization in mental health involves work with residents and institutions in the community served by the mental health agency, the community organizers and the community organization methods should have roots in, and characteristics indigenous to, the various population groups residing in the local community. Frequently, the community organizers are professionals or paraprofessionals who come from the local population subgroups. In other instances, the indigenous characteristics may be learned through study and observation (Tarail, 1979).

Technology of Marketing

Community organization skills and methods have been found to be valuable in "selling" the services of the mental health agency to the community, as well as in motivating potential clients and patients to utilize services. In this connection, community organization also has been found helpful in the development of effective political relationships with funding agencies and legislators on behalf of the facility.

At the Maimonides Community Mental Health Center committees of the community board, including in their membership community leaders from various ethnic groups, have been established to act as liaisons between the facility and the people in the community who are potential users of the service. These committees have organized parent education workshops jointly with parents' associations and have set up mental health education programs in unions, recreation centers, and churches and synagogues; frequently, the committees publish brochures, newsletters, and fliers describing the services offered by the center.

Another example, again at the Maimonides Community Mental Health Center, involves participation by community leaders in all negotiations with city, state, and federal funding agencies for funds for the mental health center. The community leaders represent tens of thousands of people who are members of organizations including trade unions, parent associations, churches, and synagogues. The government agency staff and political leaders on all levels of government generally tend to be impressed with the advocacy for the agency on the part of the community representatives, who reflect the interests of large voting constituencies (Tarail, 1972).

Building Indigenous Leadership

Community leaders are involved in diverse voluntary activities and political functions in the local community. They often are busy in schools, churches and synagogues, unions, or political clubs. Thus, it may be necessary to encourage local people with a special commitment to mental health to take on community leadership roles. Community organization methods are valuable here and should be utilized in such leadership development efforts.

Community Political Process

A pervasive problem in our society is a profound sense of hopelessness, powerlessness, and defeatism. Community organization techniques can help overcome these feelings and develop political and legislative action skills among local community groups and local community leaders. This process is essential as a base for creating constituency support for the mental health field and for the specific mental health facility (Dodson, 1966).

In this connection, community organization in mental health has demonstrated that an effective way of mobilizing people is to develop self-help movements around common needs and social change. Such movements help to offset the deep sense of helplessness and distrust regarding health and mental health services among consumers. For example, tens of thousands of senior citizens in big cities have been organized into senior citizens' councils, golden age clubs, or friendship clubs. These organizations represent the interests of senior citizens in political and legislative action and provide referral, social, educational, insurance, and other services. Workers in the field of geriatrics have found that participation in these organizations has been therapeutic to the senior citizens, preventing depression, social withdrawal, and a deep sense of being discarded and unwanted (Galiher, Needleman, and Rolfe, 1977).

At the Maimonides Community Mental Health Center a program of parent education resulted in the organization of Hispanic parents in a school with 90 percent Hispanic pupils. With the help of the community organizer, the parents' group achieved the implementation of bilingual programs and the employment of Hispanic and bilingual staff. The change in personnel and programs benefited the Hispanic children emotionally and academically.

In another program at the Maimonides Community Mental Health Center, clients in a neighborhood heavily populated by families on welfare were organized into advocacy groups. These committees of welfare clients helped each other and maximixed their ability to receive benefits and services from the local social services center. The committees also arranged single-parent mental health education and therapy groups.

Participation in the struggle to better their conditions appears to have beneficial effects on the individuals involved. Community organization technology can be used to train indigenous leaders and groups in the methods and processes of self-help. In a sense, therefore, this type of program is a primary prevention strategy and a mental health maintenance service.

Applications of Community Organization

Community organization technology and social workers trained in community organization have been involved in a number of programs and special activities at community mental health centers, family agencies, decentralized outreach clinics of state mental hospitals, and other service delivery facilities. In addition, community organization methods have been effective in health planning organizations, such as health systems agencies and federal, state, and county mental health planning organizations, and in the development of constituencies supporting national health insurance, mental retardation programs, and mental health services (especially in state hospitals). In recent years, moreover, community psychiatry, community psychology, and community mental health nursing have begun to use community organization methods (Tarail, 1971a).

Service Planning

Social work community organizers have been employed by community mental health centers and other mental health facilities and have participated in the planning of new facilities in local communities. The 1963 Community Mental Health Centers Construction Act required preliminary planning studies to identify the mental health needs of the individuals and families residing in the local community, to assess the mental health and other human services agencies serving the local community, and to specify the initial organization of representative community boards that later would govern the new mental health facility. Funds are available in the form of special planning grants from the federal government for this important planning process.

More recently, social work community organizers have been employed as key personnel in state, county, and city health planning agencies. Community organization has contributed unique skills in negotiating with and encouraging the participation of, community leaders and local human services organizations in the planning process itself, in the determination of policies and service priorities, in the conduct of needs studies, and in the identification of high-risk populations. Community organizers also have been involved in the establishment of local planning committees comprised of both providers and representatives of consumers and in the development of coordinating mechanisms for all the health, mental health, and human services agencies in the local community (Perlman and Gurin, 1972).

Community Advisory and Governing Boards

Community organizers have made vital contributions to the mandated organization of community advisory boards, composed of community leaders and consumers of mental health services, and, in the instance of freestanding community mental health centers, in the development of commmunity governing boards. The appropriate community organization technology includes methods of identifying formal and informal community leaders and the gatekeepers in the local service area; insuring the balanced representation on boards of various ethnic, age, sex, and class groups in the local community; organizing functioning committees; training community leaders for leadership on the community boards for mental health; and helping community leaders and agency administrators and clinical personnel with the operation of the new community boards (Kupst, Reidda, and McGee, 1975; Tarail, 1972).

The community board structure, mandated by federal law and regulations, represents a special problem in psychiatry and mental health, fields that in the past rarely had input and participation from community leaders and consumers of mental health services in decisionmaking on agency services. There is, in fact, a tradition of alienation from the local community on the part of mental health professionals and hospital and clinical service administrators.

The organization of community boards was complicated also by the stigma connected with mental illness and the historic downgrading of public support for mental health services in this country. In addition, community leaders needed training in mental health issues and psychiatry. Many leaders were initially suspicious, perceiving the mental health facilities as incarcerating institutions.

Community organization techniques were used to encourage attendance at community board training sessions devoted to exploring the available mental health programs and modalities of service; to set up joint committees of professional providers from the facility and community leaders responsible for evaluating mental health programs; to recruit local personnel for community mental health center staff positions; and to establish liaisons between the mental health agency and potential local consumer groups, such as parents' associations, religious organizations, youth groups, and senior citizens' groups. In many communities (both urban and rural) split into racial or ethnic groups, economic or social classes, or neighborhoods, community organization techniques focused on mental health concerns have helped bring together representatives of groups in conflict.

Mental Health Consortiums

Some of the new community mental health centers have been located on the campuses of general hospitals; others have been established as free-standing facilities in local communities. Some new comprehensive mental health agencies were developed initially as consortiums of existing mental health facilities. These consortiums usually included the local general hospital department of psychiatry, with its inpatient unit; a local family service agency; a local child guidance clinic; a local state mental hospital; a local rehabilitation agency; and so on. Consortiums frequently have been used to provide comprehensive mental health services in rural counties (e.g., the Rockland County, New York, Community Mental Health Center).

In this connection, community organization methods have been useful in developing channels for cooperation among the agencies linked in the consortium. Community organization technology has been particularly valuable in overcoming the bureaucratic self-interest and the drive to survive among the individual members of such consortiums. Community organization technology has facilitated the establishment of interagency planning and administrative committees, the delineation of specialized functions, and the development of the collaborative processes essential to the production of bylaws and policies reflecting the operation of the new comprehensive agency.

Prevention and Alternate Care Programs

Community organizers have made unique contributions to the establishment of a variety of programs aimed at the prevention of mental illness, especially in the areas of secondary and tertiary prevention (Caplan, 1971). The idea of providing services in the early stages of the development of mental health problems in individuals and families has stimulated early identification and outreach programs of various sorts. For instance, the

Maimonides Community Mental Health Center pioneered in the development of mass mental health screening programs for children.

Community organization methods have been utilized to set up formal collaborative relationships between schools and mental health agencies, establishing a foundation for effective cooperation between clinical mental health professionals and nursery schools, Headstart programs, and kindergartens for preschoolers and public and parochial schools for older children. In this connection, staff of the mental health facility contact the local superintendent of schools or local principals and arrange meetings between school personnel and the director and staff of the mental health services agency. A joint committee is established to plan mental health screening and consultation programs in the schools or other child care facilities. These school–mental health agency committees develop disposition and treatment plans for all children with mental health problems, involving the family's access to the mental health agency, curriculum changes, counseling to the parents, and often medical and social services. Community organizers also have been effective in motivating parents to arrange follow-up treatment for their children when the screening process has identified pathology (Tarail, 1971b).

Various prevention programs in mental health have been developed to serve the aged. Senior citizens usually do not utilize mental health services during the early stages of illness: they may be influenced by the social stigma connected with mental illness, or they may be fearful of psychiatric treatment, perceiving it, on the basis of experience with relatives or neighbors, as potential incarceration in mental hospitals. Community organizers on the staff of the local mental health facility have been able to make contact with senior citizen groups and other local organizations. Through such contacts, committees including representatives of the senior citizen organizations and the clinical staff of the mental health agency have been established. These committees have planned and implemented mental health education programs in the form of lectures, seminars, and workshops; mental health screening in senior citizen centers; and volunteer home companion programs for homebound aged persons. Community organizers also have been effective in stimulating the mental health agency to study the special needs of the aged and to develop more effective programs in geriatric psychiatry.

One of the important contemporary trends in the field of mental health is the development of community services that represent an alternative to hospitalization. Such systems include diagnostic and treatment outreach clinics, day/night hospitals, and the relatively new, federally funded, local community support programs for mental patients previously hospitalized in state psychiatric facilities. A number of states, including California and New York, have moved in this direction. The experience of many state hospitals and community mental health centers has demonstrated that where alternative systems of mental health service have been established and have been effectively utilized by individuals and families with severe mental health problems, the rate of hospitalization and the length of hospital stays have been substantially reduced (Task Panel on Prevention, 1978).

There is a direct relationship between this contemporary deinstitutionalization drive and the rehabilitation approaches that have been identified as part of tertiary prevention. Here the objective is to help a mentally ill person substantially improve his or her social functioning despite the limitations of the illness, which we may not know enough about scientifically at present to cure. In this connection, community organizers, in collaboration with professionals from all mental health disciplines, have been instrumental in states like California, Illinois, and New York in developing rehabilitation programs and establishing systems of coordinated services among fragmented agencies around the needs of individual clients and patients, including outpatient treatment, home care, and concrete social services involving housing, jobs, and welfare benefits (New York State Office of Mental Health, 1980).

Consultation and Education

Consultation and education programs represent one of the five major elements of service mandated by federal law for the community mental health centers now in operation (National Institute of Mental Health, 1979). Such programs also have been established by state mental hospitals, general hospital departments of psychiatry, family mental health agencies, and child psychiatry clinics. The services include consultation programs for guidance counselors, principals, teachers, and other school personnel; psychiatric consultation programs for inpatient and outpatient divisions of nonpsychiatric medical departments in general hospitals; mental health consultation services for public health department clinics; and mental health training for school personnel, police, clergy, caseworkers in county departments of social services, nonpsychiatric physicians and other medical specialists, and other non-mental health personnel working in institutions serving people with mental health problems.

In addition, community mental health education services for individuals and families residing in the catchment area include parent education workshops and seminars; premarital counseling; mental health education for senior citizens; single-parent groups; sex education; and groups of patients with serious physical problems, such as open-heart surgery patients.

The community organizer often is utilized to initiate collaboration between institutions such as schools, hospitals, churches, and police precincts and the mental health facility, with joint planning of consultation and training programs. The consultation and training programs themselves are conducted by clinicians on the staff of the mental health facility.

Local mental health facilities are using community organizers to set up indigenous consumer committees charged with developing special mental health education programs. These committees often include leaders of parent associations, senior citizen organizations, youth organizations, and religious organizations, with staff psychiatrists, psychologists, clinical social workers, and nurses providing discussion group leadership and didactic material.

Mental health community organizers also have brought the mental health agency into close working contact with block associations and business and industrial enterprises. Methods of providing services in this area range from seminars and workshops of a formal character to informal groups to radio programs. The most successful consultation and education programs have been developed as the result of joint planning by service recipients and providers.

Combating Social Stigma

A profound social stigma exists in our culture with regard to mental illness. This stigma is more pervasive than that associated with any other illness or disease. Guilt and shame often are deeply connected with mental health problems in a family, and these feelings complicate treatment. The techniques of community organization can be helpful in combating the stigma of mental illness and in motivating individuals and families to utilize their local mental health facility during the early stages of a mental health problem.

A variety of programs involving the use of community organization methods have proven effective in enhancing the utilization of mental health services despite the stigma associated with mental illness. In some community mental health centers, community organizers have set up parent education or counseling groups. These groups are organized through parent associations, church organizations, and trade unions. Under the leadership of mental health professionals, seminars and case discussions review the mental health needs of children and families. These educational, and sometimes therapeutic, groups frequently act as bridges between the parents and the mental health services and often serve as feeders into the clinical services. Similar programs have been organized for senior citizens and youth.

In other instances, community organizers have arranged for educational articles to be written by mental health professionals on the staff of the local community mental health facility and to be published in local newspapers and in-house organs of community organizations such as churches and trade unions. Emphasis is placed on minimizing the deep sense of guilt on the part of relatives about the mental illness of a family member and on interpreting the benefits of mental health services.

Community organizations methods that involve large numbers of individuals in the community in preventive programs and mental health maintenance activities often have a secondary gain in relation to the reduction of stigma. As individuals participate in such programs, their knowledge of mental health problems and therapies substantially increases, which appears to create positive attitudes toward mental health services and to correct misapprehensions about mental illness.

A stigma reduction program must reach out to all sections of the population that are not utilizing mental health services either because they do not need them or because they fear stigmatization; develop adult and youth mental health education campaigns throughout the community and in grassroots organizations of the client population; encourage participation by community organizers in in-service training and clinical conferences: develop effective primary, secondary, and tertiary prevention programs in the community served by the mental health agency; establish committees through which community leaders and potential consumers of mental health services participate in decisionmaking and in rehabilitation and reentry programs; and involve community gatekeepers in mental health education and consultation programs. The specialized knowledge and skills of community organizers are essential to the implementation of programs aimed at reducing the stigma associated with mental illness and with the utilization of mental health services on the part of local residents.

Coordination of Support Services

Community organization skills and methods have been particularly helpful in the coordination of community support services around the needs of individual clients and their families. Various mental health facilities, including mental health centers and state psychiatric hospitals, have used community organizers to develop bridges, joint conferences, and referral systems between the mental health facility and the local department of social services, local social security office, local health department, local hospital, local vocational guidance and placement service, and other local, federal, state, city, or county human service agencies. For patients discharged from state mental hospitals, community organization methods frequently are effective in bringing together the fragmented services that exist in every community into a well-coordinated and holistic support system aimed at helping the acute or chronic patient in the community move toward an appropriate level of self-sufficiency (New York State Office of Mental Health, 1980).

Local Councils of Mental Health Agencies

Community organizers on the staffs of county, city, and state departments of mental health and mental retardation and local mental health centers have established local councils of mental health and mental retardation agencies and facilities. In this connection, the workers often are called health or mental health planners. Such professionals frequently are responsible for the development of plans in relation to the mental health services in a given area, cutting across bureaucratic and funding lines. The workers also are responsible for involving providers and consumers from different sections of the geographic area in the planning process itself. Councils of mental health agencies often encourage community advocates of mental health and mental retardation services to bring the community's needs to the attention of county, city, and state legislators.

Clinical Conferences

In many centers, community organizers attend clinical conferences on patients' diagnosis and treatment, clinical staff meetings, and clinical in-service training seminars. The community organizers add an important dimension to these discussions. They are knowledgeable about social stresses that may be important components in the diagnosis and treatment of many mental health problems. Of course, in turn, the community organizer acquires insight into clinical mental health services, which enables him or her to function more effectively and to use community organization skills more appropriately in relation to the mental health service objectives of the center.

Training Clinicians, Paraprofessionals, and Community Leaders

In many mental health facilities, community organizers are involved in in-service training of clinicians from the various mental health disciplines. The community organizer can make contributions that are especially valuable in the community psychiatry components of psychiatric residents' training, community organization training for clinical social workers, and outreach and prevention training for psychiatric and mental health nurses. The principles and concepts of community organization, identified previously, should be part of the curriculum that community organization specialists teach to professional mental health personnel.

Community organizers are especially effective in training indigenous paraprofessionals, who then function as volunteer or salaried mental health workers, in community and neighborhood organization skills. Such paraprofessionals are effective bridges between the agencies and potential consumers in the local community (Tarail, 1979).

As I noted earlier, community organizers also are involved in teaching community leaders about mental health matters. They may recruit and train community leaders to participate effectively as community board members, as members of boards of visitors in state psychiatric hospitals, and as resource personnel for mental health committees requiring their input.

Outreach

Community organizers often are key workers in preparing neighborhoods for the establishment of outreach clinics, group homes for mental patients, and other outreach mental health programs. Their functions include identifying, educating, and motivating high-risk populations that traditionally have not utilized mental health services; educating and preparing neighborhood leaders for the acceptance of new outreach mental health clinics; obtaining the approval and the collaboration of neighborhood leaders in establishing group residences for mentally retarded and mentally ill persons discharged from hospitals and institutions; and establishing miniclinics in storefronts, public school buildings, churches, union halls, social service centers, shopping centers, and other local facilities.

Development of Constituencies

Community organizers are especially effective in developing community support for the mental health facility. Agency competition for funds and the need for effective legislation on city, state, and county levels require the political action of constituencies committed to helping the mental health facility survive and develop. Such organized community support has not existed in the past for mental health, as it has for education and health services (Connery, 1968). Involving community leaders in lobbying requires the political action and organization skills possessed by social workers trained in community organization. This constituency support is essential today not only for local mental health facilities but also for state, county, and city mental health departments and community service boards. In addition, community organizers can help to develop coalitions of local mental health services that work together to obtain increased government funding and more effective mental health legislation.

Trends

Deinstitutionalization: Pressure for Community Services

Under pressure from court decisions regarding the treatment of mental patients, requirements for cost-effectiveness, and the need to establish alternate systems of care, state psychiatric hospitals have moved rapidly within the past decade to discharge large numbers of mental patients. State departments of mental health throughout the country have been emphasizing community care as a substitute for hospital care. Former state hospital patients have been placed in group homes and referred to local clinics, community mental health centers, and local general hospital departments of psychiatry for treatment after discharge from the state facility.

Both the state hospitals and the local mental health agencies have had to develop, on behalf of the tens of thousands of discharged state hospital patients, local systems of integrated social, medical, and mental health services. Coordinating these programs requires the knowledge and skills of the community organizer (New York State Office of Mental Health, 1980).

Integration of Services

In all states throughout the country, and often in cities and counties, between six and eight fragmented systems of mental health services are in operation. These systems often are separate from, and in competition with, each other; most are run under different auspices; and frequently these programs have developed on an ad hoc basis. The various mental health service providers include voluntary general hospital departments of psychiatry; county and municipal hospital departments of psychiatry; community mental health centers; state psychiatric hospitals; freestanding mental health clinics, family agencies, and child guidance clinics; school and forensic psychiatric services; Veterans Administration hospital departments of psychiatry; and private practitioners (psychiatrists, psychologists, and social workers). The fragmentation of these systems tends to result in cost inefficiency and ineffective treatment programs for mental health problems.

In many states the trend is to develop integrated and unified systems of services by replanning and reordering the functions of these different facilities in local communities (New York State Office of Mental Health, 1980). States, counties, and cities also are linking agencies by using combinations of state and local staff, integrated management and administration, and client service plans that cut across agency lines. Such integrated systems are perceived to be cost-effective and highly successful in terms of service. Some of the planners and administrators in the forefront of this effort are finding community organization methods and technology helpful in the development of integrated systems of service. We may look for increased pressure from policymakers in federal and state funding and monitoring agencies for local mental health services to move in this direction during the next decade.

Implications of the Mental Health Systems Act of 1980

The Mental Health Systems Act of 1980 included provisions on the objectives, the priorities, and the funding of community mental health services for at least the next five to ten years. Briefly, the new law emphasized community mental health services; continued a program for funding and developing comprehensive community mental health centers; provided funding for holistic, biopsychosocial services in local communities for former state hospital patients; provided categorical grants for services to priority populations, such as children and youth, the aged, and the chronically mentally ill; increased the funding for nonreimbursable, nonclinical consultation, education, and preventive mental health services; and encouraged the development of unified service systems in local urban neighborhoods and in rural counties. Under this new law, community mental health agencies and facilities will have even a greater need than in the past for community organization technology.

The three trends briefly identified here—deinstitutionalization, integration of services, and emphasis on community mental health care—depend in large measure on community organization. As more positions become available for professionals who possess the skills and technology of community organization, more social workers with experience and training in this area will be employed and will make important contributions in the mental health field. Most administrators and clinical professionals in the field have little training and skill in the community organization methods essential to the implementation of the policy and program trends identified here. Schools of social work, sensitive to these trends, would do well to increase the number of social workers they graduate who are trained in community organization and who, therefore, would be most eligible for employment now and in the future in the mental health field.

Summary

Community organization strategy, process, and technology are important elements in achieving the goals of a community mental health agency. The thrust of community organization within an intervention context of social planning, is prevention, consultation, education, outreach, and planning. In addition, community organizers have been making important contributions in clinical services, in reaching high-risk populations, in overcoming the stigma connected with mental illness, in administration, in community board development, and in the community, public, and political relations essential to the survival of the local mental health facility.

While community organization recently has been included in the training of some mental health administrators, public health nurses, public health specialists, and health planners, social workers with specialized training and experience in community organization have been the primary professional group employed by the agencies to carry out the programs described in this chapter. The community mental health movement needs the special skills and processes characteristic of community organization in order to enhance the ability of mental health agencies to achieve their objectives. Thus, it is fortunate that training programs have begun to emphasize community organization in the professional education of mental health and health administrators, psychiatrists, clinical psychologists, and mental health nurses. Success in bringing mental health services to urban and rural areas throughout the country depends heavily on the availability of personnel well-trained in community organization.

REFERENCES

BRAGER, G., and SPECHT, H. (eds.). *Community Organizing.* New York: Columbia University Press, 1973.

CAPLAN, G. *Principles of Preventive Psychiatry.* New York: Basic Books, 1964.

Community Mental Health Centers Act, P.L. 88–164, P.L. 94–63, P.L. 95–622, P.L. 96–13.

CONNERY, R. H., BUCKSTROM, C. H., DENNER, D. R., FRIEDMAN, J., KROLL, M., MARDEN, R. H., McCLUSKEY, C., MEEKISON, P., and MORGAN, J. A., JR. *The Politics of Mental Health: Organizing Community Mental Health in Metropolitan Areas.* New York: Columbia University Press, 1968.

CURIEL, H., BROCHSTEIN, J. R., CHENEY, C. C., and ADAMS, G. L. "Interdisciplinary Team Teaching in a Barrio Primary Care Mental Health Setting." *Journal of Education for Social Work* 1979, *15*(3):44–50.

DODSON, D. W. "The Community Organization Worker and the Urban Encounter." *Power Conflict and Community Organizations.* New York: New York University, 1966.

FERGUSON, E. A. *Social Work: An Introduction.* Philadelphia: Lippincott, 1963.

GALIHER, C. B., NEEDLEMAN, J., and ROLFE, A. J. "Consumer Participation." In H. Rosen (ed.), *The Consumer and the Health Care System.* New York: Spectrum, 1977.

Health Policy Advisory Center. *Health Pac Bulletins,* May 1969; December 1969; May 1970; and June 1970. New York: Health Policy Advisory Center.

Joint Commission for Accreditation of Hospitals. *Guidelines and Standards for*

Ambulatory Care. Chicago: Joint Commission for Accreditation of Hospitals, 1978.

Joint Commission on Mental Illness and Health. *Action for Mental Health: Final Report of the Joint Commission on Mental Illness and Health 1961.* New York: Basic Books, 1961.

KENNEDY, J. F. "Special Message to the Congress on Mental Illness and Mental Retardation." In *Public Papers of the Presidents of the United States: John F. Kennedy . . . January 1–November 22, 1963.* Washington, D.C.: U.S. Government Printing Office, 1964.

KUPST, M., REIDDA, P., and MCGEE, T. F. "Community Mental Health Boards: A Comparison of Their Development, Functions, and Powers by Board Members and Mental Health Staff." *Community Mental Health Journal* 1975, *11*(3):249–256.

Mental Health Systems Act, P.L. 96–398, October 7, 1980.

National Institute of Mental Health. *Program Guidelines for the Community Mental Health Centers Act.* Rockville, Md.: Department of Health, Education, and Welfare, 1979.

New York State Office of Mental Health. *1981 Update: Five Year Comprehensive Plan for Mental Health Services.* Albany: New York State Office of Mental Health, 1980.

PERLMAN, R., and GURIN, A. D. *Community Organization and Social Planning.* New York: Wiley, 1972.

Task Panel on Prevention, President's Commission on Mental Health. *Task Panel Reports Submitted to the President's Commission on Mental Health,* vol. 4. Washington, D.C.: U.S. Government Printing Office, 1978.

ROTHMAN, J. "Three Models of Community Organization Practice, Their Mixing and Phasing." In F. M. Cox, J. L. Erlich, J. Rothman, and J. E. Tropman (eds.), *Strategies of Community Organization.* (3rd. ed.). Itasca., Illinois: F. E. Peacock, 1979.

SROLE, L., LANGNER, T. S., MICHAEL, S. T., OPLER, M. K., and RENNIE, T. A. C. *Mental Health in the Metropolis: The Midtown Manhattan Study.* New York: McGraw-Hill, 1962.

TARAIL, M. "Careers in Community Psychiatry: Community Psychiatry—Methods and Techniques." *Career Directions* (Sandoz Pharmaceuticals), April 1971, pp. 28–37. (a)

———. *Mental Health and Learning: A Collaborative Program between a Comprehensive Community Mental Health Center and Title I Schools.* Washington, D.C.: U.S. Government Printing Office, 1971. (b)

———. *Community Participation: Issues and Implications for Administrators.* Rockville, Md.: New York Association of Administrators, 1972.

———. "The Community Mental Health Worker: The Role and Function of Indigenous Paraprofessionals in a Comprehensive Community Mental Health Center" In S. R. Alley, Judith Blanton, and R. E. Feldman (eds.), *Paraprofessionals in Mental Health.* New York: Human Sciences, 1979.

———. *A Study and Recommendations re Administrative Training Needs of New Community Mental Health Center Directors.* Rockville, Md.: National Institute of Mental Health, 1979.

———. "Current and Future Issues in Community Mental Health." *Psychiatric Quarterly* 1980, *52*(1):27–38

PART FOUR

Some Fundamental Issues

In this section three important areas of concern for the fields of social work and mental health are presented. John S. McNeil and Roosevelt Wright, in Chapter 9, discuss the deleterious consequences of institutional racism for blacks, Hispanics, and Native Americans. Any meaningful effort to respond to the mental health needs of these Americans is contingent, in part, on understanding the relationship between racism and mental health. Sociodemographic characteristics, utilization of mental health services, representation in the core mental health professions, and mental health research are systematically considered vis-à-vis these ethnic groups.

Interdisciplinary teams are discussed by James W. Callicutt and Pedro J. Lecca in Chapter 10. They review some of the advantages and problems of interdisciplinary team practice, discuss interdisciplinary training, and consider the interdisciplinary team approach in nontraditional mental health settings.

The concluding chapter, by Joseph J. Bevilacqua and A. Levond Jones, deals with the social worker's involvement in mental health research. They note the profession's poor record in this area but point out meritorious exceptions. They also briefly look at an ongoing mental health manpower research project to give a sense of the design of an empirical study. Finally, they discuss the future of research in the context of the survival of the human services professions, including social work.

CHAPTER 9

Special Populations: Black, Hispanic, and Native American

John S. McNeil
Roosevelt Wright

THE MENTAL HEALTH and illness of the black, Hispanic, and Native American population has been the subject of much scientific and scholarly debate. Our understanding of the etiology of mental disabilities within these groups has increased during the past two decades, but there is still much to be learned. Until rather recently, our theoretical and empirical knowledge of the mental health status of black and Hispanic Americans came from a series of studies of these groups in urban settings (Lewis, 1961; Moynihan, 1965; Rainwater, 1966). Research regarding Native Americans has focused on reservation residents and those at the bottom of the socioeconomic ladder (Wax, 1971). These studies, for the most part, were conducted by white researchers who, because of their own ignorance and biases, did not evaluate accurately the sociopsychological milieu in which the subjects lived. White researchers, in fact, have in the past focused on the intrapsychic deficiencies of ethnic groups as the optimum predictors of mental disabilities. As a result, they have systematically downplayed the importance of the environmental conditions created by institutional racism. Ethnic researchers, on the other hand, focus their investigations on the environmental milieu. Their studies clearly indicate that racism functions as a major part of the etiology of much of the mental illness seen in these groups (Grier and Cobb, 1968; Smith, Burlen, Mosely, and Whitney, 1978; Willie, Kramer, and Brown, 1973).

The deleterious consequences of institutional racism extend to the self-identity, the physical and mental health, and the personality development of ethnic group members in diverse ways. Many are continually exposed to stressful life situations in which they experience severe insults to their personality (Shannon, 1973; Thomas and Sillen, 1972; Willie et al., 1973). Consequently, any meaningful effort to respond to the mental health needs of these Americans must rest on empirical understanding of the relationship between racism and mental health status (Hare, 1978).

Recently, there has been increasing recognition of the importance of culture as a requisite ingredient in the development, maintenance, and provision of mental health services in our society (Nobles, 1978; President's Commission on Mental Health, 1978). Culture is the expression of all that constitutes a people's everyday way of life:

> a people's culture is or includes the vast structures of language, behavior. . . customs, knowledge, symbols, ideas, and values which provide the people with a general design for living and patterns for interpreting reality. The cultural consciousness of a people represent the shared, symbolic, systematic and cumulative ideas, beliefs and knowledge of their historical, material, and spiritual processes. Because the cultural consciousness of a people and the values consistent with it particularly determine or help to define, select, create and recreate what is considered "real," normal, valuable, desirable, appropriate, etc. (and conversely, what is unreal, abnormal, undesirable, inappropriate, etc.) in the people's social milieu, it becomes and is a necessary variable in the formula of mental health services. (Nobles, 1979, p. 139)

Hence, culture must be the foundation of any meaningful analysis of mental health and illness.

Our society has a multitude of ethnic minority groups and the cultural influences within each group are both distinct and diverse. In this chapter, we have chosen to examine issues relating to the mental health status of black Americans, Hispanic Americans, and Native Americans. These populations possess de facto second-class status in our society. Their members' life chances have been compromised by overt and covert racism and by discrimination based on the color of their skin and the culture to which they belong. In addition, these groups are both overrepresented in the statistics on mental health and underserved or inappropriately served by the current mental health system in this country (President's Commission on Mental Health, 1978).

Some twenty million Americans suffer from mental or emotional disturbances, but fewer than one-third receive help. The statistics show that fourteen million persons need assistance who are not receiving services and that an overwhelming proportion of this group is found among the racial or ethnic minorities (President's Commission on Mental Health, 1978). Hence, it is critical that attention be given to those environmental and cultural factors that contribute to the diminished status of ethnic minority populations and their overrepresentation among the mentally ill. If prevention is to be a component of a rational mental health system, then measures to improve the quality of life for these groups is a necessary corollary (President's Commission on Mental Health, 1978).

Black Americans

Black Americans make up the largest minority group in the continental United States. More studies probably have been done of the black population than of any other group. Descriptive information of black Americans should give some idea of their mental health status. The following socio-demographic profile of the black population is intended to highlight the marginal existence of this group in our society. These statistics, while pointing to the social milieu in which the black population lives, have many implications for the mental health of this group. The status of blacks in relation to the institutions of health, education, and employment suggests the pervasiveness of institutional discrimination and the role of stressful life events in a variety of physical and mental illnesses (President's Commission on Mental Health, 1978).

Sociodemographic Characteristics

The black American population comprises approximately 12 percent of the total U.S. population—about 25.5 million individuals, or 12 million males and 13.5 million females (U.S. Bureau of the Census, 1979b). The median age for black males is 23.1 years; for black females, 24 years.

The life expectancy for black males at birth in 1974 was 62.9 years, compared to 68.9 years for white males. Similarly, life expectancy for black females in 1974 was 71.2 years, compared to 75 years for white females.

Mortality and morbidity rates for all ages and all causes is higher for blacks than for whites. Thus, blacks have higher death rates than do whites for most major diseases (hypertensive heart disease, tuberculosis, cirrhosis of the liver, and cerebrovascular disease) (Rudor and Santangelo, 1978). Infant mortality is 27.7 per 1,000 population for blacks, compared to 14.1 per 1,000 population for whites, and within the black population the mortality rate for male infants continues to exceed that for female infants (*Urban Research Review,* 1980).

A high incidence of poverty, job discrimination, large families, inferior education, and prejudice all act to depress the black median income (Ozawa, 1972). Almost one-third (1.6 million, or 28.2 percent) of black families were below the poverty level in 1977, compared to 7 percent (3.5 million) of white families. This figure reached 51 percent for black female heads of household, compared to 25 percent for white families in a comparable situation (*Urban Research Review,* 1980).

The median income for black families has been steadily increasing because of, among other things, the increasing proportion of black wives who work (the median income of black families whose head worked full-time year-round in 1967 was $9,349; in 1969 it was $10,635; and in 1974 it was

$12,136). However, the median income of black families relative to white families has declined since 1970. The median income ratio of black to white families was .58 in 1974; it was .61 in 1979 (President's Commission on Mental Health, 1978).

Black adults have been making significant educational gains during the past four decades but still lag behind their white counterparts. In 1940, for example, 11 percent of black men and women between the ages of 25 and 34 had completed 4 years of high school or more, compared to 39 percent of whites in this same age category. In 1975, this figure had increased to 69 percent for blacks, compared to 82 percent for whites. The median schooling completed by blacks in 1975 was 12.4 years, compared to 12.8 for whites. Additionally, in 1975 about 11 percent of black men and women 25–34 years old had completed 4 years or more of college, compared to 22 percent of whites in this age group. In 1977, approximately 21 percent of black men and women 18–24 years old were enrolled in college, compared with approximately 27 percent of white young adults (U.S. Bureau of the Census, 1979b). The proportion of blacks enrolled in institutions of higher learning remained stable between 1976 and 1978 but exceeded the 1970 level. Clearly, the smaller number of blacks with adequate preparation for employment contributes to their depressed social and economic status (*Urban Research Review,* 1980).

The economic recovery and growth experienced by the nation since the 1973–1975 recession has not been shared fully by the black population. Since 1975, blacks have made gains in the number employed (e.g., 750,000 blacks obtained new jobs between 1975 and 1977); however, black unemployment levels have remained essentially unchanged (*Urban Research Review,* 1980; U.S. Bureau of the Census, 1979b). The overall unemployment rate for black persons sixteen years of age and older in 1978 was 12 percent, compared to a 4.5 percent rate for whites sixteen years and older. In the sixteen to nineteen age bracket, the unemployment rates were 37 percent for blacks and 14 percent for whites; among men twenty years of age and over the unemployment rate for blacks in 1978 was 9.1 percent versus 5.2 percent for whites (*Urban Research Review,* 1980). Not counting persons sixteen to twenty-one years old, the overall unemployment rate for blacks in January 1978 was 11 percent and approximately 6 percent for whites.

The differential involvement of blacks and whites in the various categories of the work force is another indicator of their depressed economic status. In 1977, the proportions of black men and women employed in white-collar jobs (professional, managerial, sales, and clerical occupations) were 23 and 44 percent, respectively. The proportions of white men and women in white-collar jobs in 1977 were 40 and 61 percent, respectively. The majority (58 percent) of black men were found in blue-collar jobs. White men, however, were more likely to be found in equal percentages in white- and blue-collar jobs; estimated rates were 40 and 43 percent, respectively (U.S.

Bureau of the Census, 1979b). More than one-third (37 percent) of black women held jobs as service workers, compared to one-fifth (16 percent) of white women. These statistics demonstrate all too well that blacks continue to lag behind whites in the proportion holding high-status jobs that provide adequate pay, good benefits, and stability. Blacks are condemned to less skilled, lower paying jobs, characterized by high turnover and discrimination.

In 1978, there were 5.8 million black families. Most of them followed the nuclear family model. The period from 1975 to 1978 saw a rise in the proportion of black families maintained by a single parent and a corresponding decline in the proportion of two-parent families. Two-parent families declined from 61 percent to 56 percent of all black families during this period, while the proportion of women maintaining families alone increased from 35 to 39 percent (U.S. Bureau of the Census, 1979b). Among whites, however, two-parent families constituted 86 percent of all families. We do not mean to suggest that single-parent families per se are less conducive to mental health than are other familial types. However, we would argue, as others do, that families that do not conform to the norm (i.e., the nuclear prototype) can influence positively the mental health and functioning of their members in unique ways (Billingsley, 1968). Mental health practitioners must recognize that single-parent families usually command fewer economic and social resources, which may make them less able adequately to fulfill the needs of family members. Members of these families are therefore more vulnerable to various mental illnesses. However, we strongly argue that environmental influences such as individual and institutional patterns of racism and stressful conditions of living are the most important cause of mental illness among blacks and not the structural arrangement of their families.

Mental Health Risk

The 1960s and 1970s produced a substantial body of research on the linkages between race and mental illness (Fisher, 1969; Fried, 1969; Warheit, Holyer, and Arey, 1976). Some scholars have argued that rates of mental illness are higher for blacks than whites (Balah, 1970; Gorwitz, 1966). Others have suggested that treated mental illness rates are higher for whites than blacks (See and Miller, 1973). And finally, some have suggested that evidence concerning the differential rates of mental illness between blacks and whites is inconclusive (Warheit et al., 1976). For example, the President's Commission on Mental Health (1978), reviewing diverse methodological approaches to the study of mental illness among racial groups, concluded that as research comparing Black and White incidence and prevalence of serious mental disorder accumulated, it became clear that few certain epidemiological patterns could be identified. Recent findings continue to reflect this ambiguity. Moreover, since no recent study has attempted to determine true prevalence or incidence, it is still not known whether Blacks and Whites have similar or different rates of serious mental disorder. (P. 829)

These contradictory findings should be kept in mind throughout the following discussion.

In 1970, the overall rate of institutionalization was 41 percent higher among blacks than whites (the rate of institutionalization per 100,000 population was 1,412.7 for blacks versus 1,004.3 for whites) (Cannon and Locke, 1977). There was considerable divergence by type of institution. For example, blacks exceeded whites in mental institutions by 52 percent in 1970; in correctional institutions by about 900 percent; and in juvenile delinquency facilities by approximately 400 percent. A major reason for these disparities is that institutional racism initially directs blacks into penal institutions rather than mental health facilities. The opposite is true for whites exhibiting similar behavioral problems (Cannon and Locke, 1977).

Available data on differential use of psychiatric facilities by blacks and whites indicate that the utilization rates for blacks exceed those for whites by 45 percent. Census data show that in 1971 the utilization rate for inpatient psychiatric services was 566.8 admissions per 100,000 population for whites, compared to 806.1 admissions per 100,000 population for nonwhites or blacks. Similarly, the utilization rates for outpatient psychiatric services was 606.4 admissions per 100,000 population for whites versus 890.4 admissions per 100,000 population for blacks (Cannon and Locke, 1977). Also of interest is the relationship between admission rates to outpatient mental health facilities by race with respect to family income. Cannon and Locke (1977) reported that almost one-third of the whites and over half of the nonwhites had family incomes of less than $3,000 annually; the median family income of white admissions was almost twice that of nonwhite admissions, with the greatest disparity between white and nonwhite females.

In 1975 blacks comprised approximately 11 percent of the U.S. resident population yet accounted for 22 percent of all inpatient admissions to public mental hospitals. Admission rates among blacks (344 per 100,000 population) to state and county mental hospitals were double those of whites (161 per 100,000 population), and the racial disparity was greater between males than between females (Table 9.1). The median age of white males admitted to public mental hospitals was about four years higher than for black males, while there was no difference in median age of black and white females at time of admission (Cannon and Locke, 1977). In addition, Table 9.1 indicates that black males consistently show the highest rates of hospital admissions.

As is the case with inpatient psychiatric services, the use of outpatient services is not distributed uniformly across racial groups (Table 9.2). The

TABLE 9.1

Age Specific and Age Adjusted Rates per 100,000 Population of Outpatient Clinic Admissions, by Race and Sex, 1975

Age on Admission	White			Black		
	Both Sexes	Male	Female	Both Sexes	Male	Female
Total admissions	296,151	190,788	150,363	86,367	53,646	29,721
Age Composition, All ages	161.1	214.2	111.2	344.2	469.5	232.2
Under 18	31.6	39.3	23.6	77.8	103.1	52.2
18–24	234.0 [6]	892.1	241.8			
25–44	270.2	349.3	194.2	688.3	1032.7	406.3
45–64	213.4	276.0	155.7	414.1	412.2	413.7
65 and over	85.3	130.9	54.0	171.9	210.8	143.7
Median age	35.2	34.3	37.3	32.1	30.0	38.0
Age adjusted rate*	159.7	213.2	110.0	367.3	509.4	248.5

Source: President's Commission on Mental Health, 1978

*Adjustment based on distribution of U.S. civilian population in July 1975.

TABLE 9.2
Age Specific and Age Adjusted Rates per 100,000 Population of Outpatient Clinic Admissions, by Race and Sex, 1975

Age on Admission	White			Black		
	Both Sexes	Male	Female	Both sexes	Male	Female
Total admissions	1,171,196	528,794	642,402	198,965	90,082	108,833
Under 18	505.6	620.7	385.4	715.1	947.3	480.4
18–24	883.9	798.3	965.5	782.6	881.3	699.0
25–44	1022.1	810.3	1225.4	1407.4	931.7	1795.5
45–64	444.4	376.1	507.5	431.7	371.8	483.0
65 and over	217.9	129.2	278.9	480.9	132.9	735.0
Median age	28.5	25.0	30.7	26.1	17.8	30.0
Age adjusted rate*	639.2	587.7	682.7	813.4	730.5	865.9

Source: President's Commission on Mental Health, 1978
*Adjustment based on distribution of U.S. civilian population in July 1975.

rates of utilization of outpatient psychiatric service (e.g., public hospital outpatient clinics and community mental health centers) are consistently higher for blacks across all age groups than for whites. The admission rate for black females is relatively low until the age bracket twenty-four to forty-four, when it increases dramatically.

Table 9.3 shows the five leading diagnoses among persons admitted to state and county mental hospitals in 1975. Alcohol disorders and schizophrenia were the most frequently reported diagnoses among all males; however, alcohol disorders were first among white males and schizophrenia first among black males (Cannon and Locke, 1977). In addition, for both disorders the rates for black males were significantly higher than the rates for white males. The most frequently reported diagnosis for females was schizophrenia, with black females showing a considerably higher rate than their white counterparts. Schizophrenia was followed by alcohol disorders among black females and depressive disorders among white females (Table 9.3).

Data on the leading diagnoses for discharge from general hospital psychiatric inpatient services indicate that among both white males and females, depressive disorders rank as the most frequently reported diagnosis, followed by schizophrenia (65.3 and 131.3 per 100,000, respectively) (Table 9.4). Among both male and female blacks, however, the most frequently reported diagnosis at discharge is schizophrenia (119.3 and 117.8 per 100,000 population, respectively), followed by alcohol disorders among black males and depressive disorders among black females.

The preceding statistics indicate that among patients treated in mental health facilities whites are most likely to be diagnosed with depressive disorders while blacks are most likely to be diagnosed schizophrenic (Cannon and Locke, 1977); depression is generally regarded as a more acute than chronic illness, with a better prognosis than schizophrenia has:

> The hesitancy to diagnose Blacks as affectively ill or depressed is overly compensated for by a strong tendency to diagnose Blacks as schizophrenic more frequently than Whites. Such diagnostic differences found between Blacks and Whites could be a reflection of the diagnostic habits of psychiatrists or could be due to differences in the quality of communication between Negro patients and White psychiatrists as compared to White patients and White psychiatrists. (Cannon and Locke, 1977, p. 424)

Utilization of Mental Health Services

America's goal of adequate mental health care for black people has yet to be attained. Many of the problems in achieving this goal have to do with the agencies and organizations that comprise the various systems responsible for delivering mental health services. These organizations have heretofore been unresponsive and insensitive to the specific mental health needs of the black population (President's Commission on Mental Health, 1978):

TABLE 9.3
Five Leading Diagnoses for Admissions to State and County Hospitals, by Race, Sex, and Rate per 100,000 Population, 1975

White Male		Black Male	
Alcohol disorders	79.5	Schizophrenia	197.1
Schizophrenia	56.3	Alcohol disorders	122.0
Depressive disorders	21.7	Personality disorders	35.6
Personality disorders	16.9	Organic brain syndromes	27.0
Drug disorders	10.0	Adjustment reaction and behavior disorder—children	22.6

White Female		Black Female	
Schizophrenia	42.8	Schizophrenia	118.2
Depressive disorders	231.0	Alcohol disorders	50.1
Alcohol disorders	12.4	Organic brain syndromes	17.3
Organic brain syndromes	7.8	Depressive disorders	10.2
Personality disorders	6.6	Adjustment reaction—adult	9.8

Source: President's Commission on Mental Health, 1978

TABLE 9.4
Five Leading Diagnoses for Discharges from General Hospital Psychiatric Inpatient Services, by Race, Sex, and Rate per 100,000 Population, 1975

White Male		Black Male	
Depressive disorders	65.3	Schizophrenia	119.3
Schizophrenia	48.6	Alcohol disorders	24.7
Alcohol disorders	25.7	Depressive disorders	20.2
Personality disorders	15.2	Transient situational personality disorders	13.9
Neuroses	13.1	Personality disorders	12.4

White Female		Black Female	
Depressive disorders	131.3	Schizophrenia	117.8
Schizophrenia	54.1	Depressive disorders	68.1
Neuroses	18.1	Neuroses	15.9
Personality disorders	14.1	Drug disorders	14.1
Transient situational personality disorders	14.6	Transient situational personality disorders	13.0

Source: President's Commission on Mental Health, 1978

A major problem in health care involves the mental-health caretaker's attitude toward minority clients. Frequently, minority clients are made aware of their "second-class status" through the many contacts they must make in the agency—from intake to caseworker to therapist. The myths and stereotypes these staff persons have learned and exhibit toward minority clients lead to distrust and often inhibit success in the therapy situation. (Smith et al., 1978, p. 117)

In discussing the organizational and professional problems in delivering services to black people, the President's Commission on Mental Health (1978), indicated that the reason blacks and other minorities do not avail themselves of physical and mental health services is not lack of desire for services so much as the attitude of the health care givers. Moreover, the Commission identified other factors that discourage blacks from availing themselves of health care services:

lack of awareness of the availability of such services; the reliance on traditional media to inform Black and poor people of the existence of such services; inadequate transportation to and from health delivery agencies; and scheduled hours that are more convenient for the health delivery personnel rather than for the potential Black consumer. (President's Commission on Mental Health, 1978, p. 836)

A related problem is that the mental health needs of black people suffer the same lack of understanding on the part of the professional care giver as do other social problems faced by blacks (Willie et al., 1973). Professional health care personnel in general are trained in the traditional psychological constructs and techniques for dealing with mental illness; many of these professionals are not prepared to deal with the realities of ghetto life, which are often determinants of the behavior exhibited by blacks (Smith et al., 1978). Funnye (1970) strongly criticized human service professionals for their failure to recognize the importance of race and racism in their work with black clients.

Social work theory still insists that the sociopsychological environment of Black Americans is the same as—or is certainly only a shade different from—the environment of White Americans. In spite of the continuous bombardment of hostility heaped on Blacks solely because they are Black (in addition to all the normal pressures of life), most social work theorists persist in contending that Blacks do not develop some unique responses or do not have different needs or psychic requirements from Whites. (P. 10)

Practitioners must explore the possibility of expanding their middle-class orientations, traditional treatment modalities, and theoretical perspectives of personality to include such variables as race and ethnicity, culture, and racism. Then and only then can mental health workers look forward to a more comprehensive understanding of the mental health status of black people.

Another problem in the delivery of mental health services to blacks involves linguistic differences between black consumers and nonblack practitioners. A number of researchers have documented the differences between whites and blacks in the area of expression (both verbal and nonverbal) and the role of language as a tool for dealing with racism (Carkhuff and Pierce, 1967; Jones, 1974; Jones and Jones, 1970; Willie et al., 1974). Blacks have developed a unique communication system as a means of survival in a racist society (Smith et al., 1978). Black dialect (e.g., jive talk) has become a symbol of unity among blacks and has been used to thwart the efforts of whites to understand black behavior. The aforementioned studies suggest that most white practitioners are ill equipped to communicate effectively with black consumers. Yet white practitioners in helping situations have tended to view black-white communication problems as inhering in the client and have taken little responsibility for overcoming a major barrier to problem-solving.

A fourth problem area is related more specifically to community mental health agencies. To have an impact on the mental health problems of a particular community, the agency must have a thorough knowledge of the cultural, environmental, and economic factors peculiar to that community (Mayfield, 1972; Smith et al., 1978). These organizations must be sensitive and responsive to the problems that affect the day-to-day lives of community residents. To enhance cooperation between the mental health agency and the consumer population, mental health personnel must be willing, trained, and flexible enough to tap all the resources available in the community—health, economic, educational, and social—to meet not only the intrapsychic needs of their clients but also those externally manifested needs (Smith et al., 1978).

Finally, the high turnover rate among staff in mental health organizations and a severe shortage of trained professionals (psychiatrists, psychologists, social workers) in direct service delivery present formidable problems to the utilization of and access to mental health services by black people. Research in the social sciences has repeatedly found that methodologies and techniques prove most effective when there is status similarity or equivalence between the recipient of service and the deliverer of that treatment (Bestman, 1978; Cole, 1977). Harrison (1975), in a systematic review of thirty-two studies on the race of the therapist, corroborated the findings reported by Cole (1977) and Bestman (1978). He concluded that clients do prefer counselors of the same race; this was especially true for blacks. More important, the language elaboration of black clients was more extensive in the presence of blacks than in the presence of whites (i.e., blacks appear to talk more in the presence of other blacks). Gardner (1972), in a study on the differential effects of race, education, and experience in helping situations, reported that after one interview black clients gave higher effectiveness ratings to black therapists than to white therapists. Hence, it would be reasonable to assume that when client and practitioner are of the same race, or share similar lifestyles and value systems, there is a greater probability that the client will respond favorably to a treatment (Cole, 1977; Gardner, 1972; President's Commission on Mental Health, 1978).

It is possible to reverse the pattern of underutilization of mental health services. Personnel at the Family and Individual Services Agency in Fort Worth, Texas, were concerned that black clients were not using their services. The agency office was located in an area populated primarily by middle-class white families. Staff were almost all white. A decision was made to establish a satellite office in a predominantly black neighborhood and to staff it with a black social worker and a black clerical person. A vigorous outreach program was initiated. Within one year staff had to be increased and local residents were utilizing all available appointment hours.

Status of Mental Health Research

In terms of the amount and variety of research on blacks in the United States, there is no shortage of information. The problem is one of point of view or focus of that research (President's Commission on Mental Health, 1978). Gary (1974) identified certain deficiencies in much of the research by nonblack investigators on problems confronting the black community:

1. the white middle-class behavior norms against which black behavior is evaluated
2. the failure to take account of the interrelated forces that create and maintain racism and hence influence black mental health, and the corollary that problems of blacks are to be found within themselves and their life experiences
3. the tendency to assume the uniformity of the black experience and a propensity to focus on the lowest income groups among blacks
4. the tendency to blame the victim

Marked by these deficiencies, our knowledge about the mental health problems of black Americans is biased and skewed. We still do not have systematic, adequate data regarding both the incidence and prevalence of mental disorders among black populations and the differential utilization of mental health facilities by blacks and whites; similarly, treatment outcomes and community mental health needs have not been determined by race on a national, regional, and local basis (Cannon and Locke, 1977).

Until recently, research careers have been virtually closed to blacks. More emphasis must be given to attracting trained and competent black mental health workers to research careers. Black researchers must be allowed the opportunity to take a more active role in defining the research strategies for solving the problems and developing the resources of the black community. It is crucial that black researchers raise questions concerning the conceptual, theoretical, ethical, and methodological bases of research related to mental health issues and their application to the black community (Cannon and Locke, 1977; President's Commission on Mental Health, 1978).

Black communities in recent years have become hostile to white researchers. They feel that such research rarely results in actions beneficial to their community or individual well-being. To lessen this resistance future research should be directed toward improving understanding, changing attitudes, and creating a healthier mental health environment.

Representation in the Core Mental Health Professions

Given the documented need for mental health services among the black population, it is essential that the number of black professional and para-professional mental health practitioners be increased significantly. The supply of these workers continues to lag grossly behind the increasing demand for services (President's Commission on Mental Health, 1978). In addition, more black persons must be recruited and trained to assume administrative and managerial positions in mental health programs designed to serve largely black populations.

The President's Commission on Mental Health (quoting Cannon and Locke) published recent data on the number of blacks in the four core mental health professions:

Psychiatry: A national survey of psychiatrists was conducted by the American Psychiatric Association under contract from NIMH. Of 15,543 individuals responding to the race/ethnicity question, 226 (1.5 percent) were Black. A survey of residents in training conducted by the American Medical Association in 1973–1974 showed that in that year 82 out of 4,903 (1.7 percent) residents in psychiatry and child psychiatry were Black U.S. citizens.

Psychology: A survey of psychologists conducted by the American Psychological Association in 1972 showed that of 26,741 APA members and non-members who answered the question on race/ethnicity, 396 (1.5) percent were Black. In 1973, of the 4,796 individuals who were awarded doctoral degrees in the social sciences, including psychology, 87 or 1.8 percent were Black.

Psychiatric Nursing: There [are] no data regarding the racial/ethnic distribution of psychiatric nurses. At the time of the 1970 census, Blacks comprised 7.2 percent of all employed registered nurses. The Division of Nursing, the Department of Health, Education, and Welfare estimated that 5 percent of all registered nurses within the United States are Black. Enrollment data show that the percent of Blacks enrolled in Baccalaureate Nursing programs has grown slowly from 4.2 percent in 1962–63 to 8.5 percent in 1971–72.

Social Work: A 1975 survey of National Association of Social Workers members found that of 32,706 respondents to the race/ethnicity question, 2,486

(7.6 percent) were Black. Enrollment data show that of 17,388 full-time degree students enrolled in U.S. graduate schools of Social Work in November of 1975, 2,149 (12.4 percent) were Black. (Pp. 841–42)

In social work, the enrollment figures have been decreasing steadily; in 1976, 11.0 percent; in 1977, 10.3 percent; in 1979, 9.9 percent (*Statistics on Social Work Education in the United States*; 1975, 1976, 1977, 1979).

Summary

The preceding discussion has attempted to present a broad overview of the mental health status of the black population. The analysis leads to several important conclusions. First, individual and institutional racism not only acts as a barrier to quality mental health services for blacks but also functions as a major cause of much of the observed mental illness in this group. Second, in terms of the amount and variety of research on blacks in the United States, there is no shortage of information. Nevertheless, there is a serious shortage of mental health research from the perspective of the black researcher. Third, there is a need for a more comprehensive mental health delivery system that is sensitive to the unique cultural characteristics of the black population. Last, there is a critical need for more trained black professionals in the mental health field.

In order to improve the delivery of mental health services to the black population, it is important that we consider the mental health status of blacks in the context of environmental, cultural, and societal conditions, rather than focusing solely on the individual's intrapsychic problems. Such a shift in focus will entail modifying the traditional approaches to treating blacks, conducting mental health research, and training mental health professionals (Smith et al., 1978).

Hispanic Americans

Hispanics account for a sizable proportion of the population in the United States, but estimates vary considerably. Census figures are thought to be very conservative and therefore to represent a significant undercount. The 1973 census indicated that there were 9.6 million persons of Spanish origin in the United States (U.S. Bureau of Census, 1973). In 1980 this figure was 14.6 million (U.S. Bureau of the Census, 1981). The Hispanic population, on the basis of these figures, represented less than 8 percent of the population. Estimates that consider factors such as undocumented immigration, high fertility rates, and census undercount place the number of Hispanics who reside in the United States at more than 23 million persons. There is considerable agreement that persons of Spanish origin are the fastest growing ethnic group in the United States. Macias (1977) projected that by the year 2000 the Hispanic American population will total 55 million.

This population of Hispanic Americans includes persons from various countries (Table 9.5): Mexican Americans represent 50 percent of the total; Puerto Ricans constitute the next largest group (15 percent); about 7 percent are of Central or South American origin (1978). Hispanics, therefore, are a heterogeneous group that differs in significant ways from the Anglo population.

Sociodemographic Characteristics

One of the most critical sociodemographic variants is language. Traditionally, Americans have been monolingual and have tended to demand that all immigrants and visitors speak English. Individuals who do not have a command of English are looked upon askance and at times disparaged. However, 70 percent of Hispanics indicate that Spanish is their mother tongue and more than half speak primarily Spanish at home; many prefer to speak Spanish. Approximately 20 percent report difficulty with English (President's Commission on Mental Health, 1978).

Hispanic Americans tend to live in large metropolitan areas, such as Los Angeles, Chicago, and New York. One of four families in the general population lives in the central city of a metropolitan area, whereas half the families of Spanish origin live in these locations.

Hispanic Americans are also the youngest of all the ethnic groups, with a median age of 20.7 years, compared to a median age of 28.6 for the general population. Furthermore, 14 percent of all Puerto Ricans and Mexicans are under 5 years of age, in contrast to slightly less than 8 percent of the

TABLE 9.5
Hispanic Population, by Origin, 1978

	Number (in thousands)	Percent
Total Spanish origin	12,046	100.0
Mexican	7,151	59.4
Puerto Rican	1,823	15.1
Cuban	689	5.7
Central or South American	863	7.2
Other	1,519	12.6

Source: U.S. Bureau of the Census, 1979a.

general population. This lower median age may reflect the previously mentioned high fertility rate and/or the lower life expectancy of Hispanics. In fact, minorities have a life expectancy that is 6 years less than that for whites (U.S. Department of Health, Education, and Welfare, 1977).

The higher fertility rate for Hispanics can again be seen when we compare family size. Hispanics are twice as likely to belong to families that have seven or more members and over one-third of these large families have incomes that place them below the poverty line (President's Commission on Mental Health, 1978). A disproportionate number of all Hispanics are included in the poverty population, approximately 12 percent, whereas they acount for only 4.5 percent of the general population (U.S. Department of Health, Education, and Welfare, 1977). These data become more meaningful when the figures are broken down by specific Hispanic groups (Table 9.6). Families of Mexican origin tend to be larger than those of other Hispanic groups, with Puerto Rican families ranking second and Cubans having the smallest families of the three groups.

Intergroup comparisons among Hispanics also show differences in income. Cubans have the highest median family income, the fewest families with earnings below the poverty line, and the largest number of families with an annual income in excess of $15,000 (Table 9.7).

Padillo, Ruiz, and Alvarez (1975) described the "culture of poverty" of people of Spanish origin. Several factors combine to create the culture: low income, unemployment, underemployment, undereducation, poor housing, prejudice and discrimination, cultural and linguistic barriers, and

---

TABLE 9.6
Hispanic Families, by Origin and Family Size, 1978

Family Size	Total Spanish	Mexican	Puerto Rican	Cuban	Other Spanish*	Not of Spanish Origin†
All families (in thousands)	2,764	1,623	437	186	518	54,451
Percent	100.0	100.0	100.0	100.0	100.0	100.0
Two persons	23.9	21.4	24.3	30.1	29.2	39.2
Three persons	23.0	21.3	22.3	24.7	28.4	22.0
Four persons	22.6	22.7	24.1	26.3	19.9	20.5
Five persons	14.8	15.8	17.3	7.5	12.0	10.8
Six persons	7.9	9.5	5.8	5.4	5.4	4.5
Seven or more persons	7.8	9.4	6.2	5.4	5.2	3.0
Mean number of persons	3.88	4.06	3.78	3.51	3.55	3.31

Source: U.S. Bureau of the Census, 1979a.
*Includes Central or South American origin and other Spanish origin.
†Includes families maintained by persons who did not know or did not report on origin.

TABLE 9.7
Income of Hispanic Families, by Origin, 1977

	Median Family Income	Percent of Families with Income below $4,000	Percent of Families with Income of $15,000 or More
Total Spanish origin	$11,421	10.4	34.7
Mexican	11,742	9.1	34.9
Puerto Rican	7,972	16.1	24.4
Cuban	14,182	8.9	46.5
Central or South American	11,280	10.4	37.7
Other	12,855	9.9	39.4
Not of Spanish origin*	16,284	6.1	54.9

Source: U.S. Bureau of the Census, 1979a.
*Includes families maintained by persons who did not know or did not report on origin.

powerlessness. After racism, educational opportunity is probably the most important factor predictive of poverty (Table 9.8):

> Persons of Spanish origin in the United States have not yet reached the educational attainment level of non-Spanish persons. By March 1978, about 17 percent of all persons of Spanish origin 25 years old and over had completed less than 5 years of school; the corresponding proportion for non-Spanish persons was 3 percent. Also, only 41 percent of Spanish persons 25 years old and over had completed 4 years of high school or more, compared with 67 percent of the non-Spanish population in that age group. However, recent gains have been made in educational attainment for persons of Spanish origin. Although only 17 percent of Spanish-origin persons 65 years old and over reported in March 1978 having completed 4 years of high school or more, about 57 percent of Spanish persons 25 to 29 years old had completed 4 years of high school or more. Within the Spanish population, persons of Cuban origin had a significantly higher educational level than persons of Mexican or Puerto Rican origin. Only 9 percent of Cubans 25 years old and over had completed less than 5 years of school, yet 23 percent of Mexican-origin persons, and 15 percent of Puerto Ricans in that age group had completed less than 5 years of school. Furthermore, 49 percent of Cuban-origin persons had completed 4 years of high school or more, compared to 34 percent of those of Mexican origin, and 36 percent of those of Puerto Rican origin. (U.S. Bureau of the Census, 1979a, p. 6)

Hispanics have a much higher unemployment rate than do whites and are congregated in the lower paying jobs. Moreover, earnings among Hispanic males are consistently below those of males of non-Spanish origin.

TABLE 9.8
Percentage of the Hispanic Population Twenty-five Years Old and Over, by Years of Schooling, Origin, and Age, 1978

Years of Schooling and Age	Total Spanish	Mexican	Puerto Rican	Cuban	Other Spanish*	Not of Spanish Origin†
Percent completed less than 5 years of school						
Total 25 years and over	17.2	23.1	15.0	9.3	5.9	3.0
25–29	5.7	7.6	4.3	(B)††	1.0	.6
30–34	9.6	12.6	8.2	(B)	3.5	.6
35–44	11.2	15.9	12.4	2.2	1.7	1.1
45–64	24.9	34.3	23.0	10.2	9.3	2.7
65 and over	45.0	65.4	(B)	20.5	19.2	8.7
Percent completed 4 years of high school or more						
Total 25 years and over	40.8	34.3	36.0	49.1	58.5	67.1
25–29	56.6	51.3	52.1	(B)	74.5	87.1
30–34	50.1	44.1	43.7	(B)	67.8	84.4
35–44	44.2	37.2	35.2	57.8	62.7	76.9
45–64	30.3	21.4	26.0	40.9	51.1	62.7
65 and over	17.3	7.1	(B)	34.9	28.3	38.6
Percent completed 4 years of college or more						
Total 25 years and over	7.1	4.3	4.2	13.9	13.8	16.1

Source: U.S. Bureau of the Census, 1979a.
*Includes Central or South American origin and other Spanish origin.
†Includes persons who did not know or did not report on origin.
††Under seventy-five thousand in this category.

Even in government jobs, Hispanics earn less than non-Hispanics. Occupational level and income are shown in Table 9.9.

Hispanics live in crowded conditions three times more frequently than do whites and are twice as likely to occupy residences with inadequate plumbing (U.S. Department of Health, Education, and Welfare, 1977). Because many Hispanics live in inner-city neighborhoods, they are among the first to be affected by urban renewal programs. Discriminatory housing practices prevent moves into better neighborhoods (Padillo and Ruiz, 1973). This culture of poverty predisposes Hispanics to "inordinate life stresses," thereby increasing the potential need for mental health services (Karno and Edgerton, 1969).

TABLE 9.9
Median Earnings of Civilians Fourteen Years Old and Over with Earnings, by Origin, Longest Held Job, Class of Worker in Longest Held Job, and Sex, 1977

Occupation and Class of Worker	Male Spanish Origin	Male Not of Spanish Origin*	Female Spanish Origin	Female Not of Spanish Origin*
Total with earnings	8,271	11,237	4,122	4,703
Occupation				
Professional, technical, and				
kindred workers	13,666	16,275	8,854	9,170
Self-employed	(B)†	22,362	(B)	2,146
Salaried	13,635	16,023	8,813	9,470
Managers and administrators,				
except farm	13,100	16,943	(B)	7,788
Self-employed	(B)	11,277	(B)	2,350
Salaried	14,352	17,897	(B)	8,385
Sales workers	9,532	11,767	3,045	2,415
Clerical and kindred workers	7,360	11,077	5,152	6,090
Craft and kindred workers	10,117	12,440	(B)	5,533
Operatives, including transport	8,500	10,212	4,776	5,145
Manufacturing	8,857	10,503	5,022	5,483
Other	8,114	9,901	3,700	3,506
Laborers, excluding farm	6,790	4,378	(B)	2,948
Farmers and farm managers	(B)	4,306	(B)	751
Farm laborers and				
supervisors	4,500	1,686	982	829
Service workers, except				
private household	6,119	4,996	2,688	2,456
Private household workers	(B)	573	1,004	726
Class of worker				
Private wage or salary workers	8,083	11,163	4,170	4,479
In agriculture	4,711	2,415	1,096	940
Not in agriculture	8,561	11,500	4,436	4,548
Government wage or				
salary workers	9,596	12,844	4,343	6,846
Public administration	12,080	15,115	(B)	7,617
Other government workers	8,563	11,363	4,251	6,566
Self-employed workers	8,429	8,538	(B)	1,801
In nonagricultural				
industries	8,614	10,284	(B)	1,801
Unpaid family workers	(B)	(B)	(B)	874

Source: U.S. Bureau of the Census, 1979a.
*Includes persons who did not know or did not report on origin.
†Under seventy-five thousand in this category.

Mental Health Risk

Assessing mental health risk is at best grossly inexact. Some indicators, however, are available, including prison and arrest statistics, mental hospital admission rates, and data on substance abuse.

Admission rates to state and county mental hospitals show a pattern that may be somewhat unexpected in view of the hypothesized link between mental illness and inordinate life stresses. Hispanics have an admission rate 50 percent lower than do other minority groups and 15 percent lower than do whites. Table 9.10 presents these rates, revealing some interesting reversals at certain age levels.

As Table 9.10 shows, at each age level, except fourteen through twenty-four, the Hispanic admission rate is lowest of the three ethnic categories. The increase for Hispanics aged fourteen through twenty-four may reflect the high level of substance abuse (drugs) among this group. Cuellar (1978) reported that in 1976 Mexican Americans diagnosed as having drug abuse problems were overrepresented in Texas state mental hospitals.

Admissions by diagnostic category are shown in Table 9.11. In 1972, approximately three in ten Hispanics admitted to mental hospitals had a diagnosis of schizophrenia, a rate substantially lower than that for other nonwhites. Alcohol and drug disorders accounted for the next two largest admission diagnostic categories for Hispanics.

Data on the experience of Hispanics with the criminal justice system must be interpreted cautiously. These data may be biased either by the statistical reporting procedures themselves or by the political and cultural values of the entire criminal justice system. Data collected in one geographic area are not readily generalizable to the entire country or to all Hispanic groups. A recent study in New York State indicated that Hispanics are ov-

TABLE 9.10
Admissions per 100,000 Population to State and County Mental Hospitals, by Age and Ethnicity, 1972

Age	Total	Hispanic	White	Other Minority
Under 14	12.7	5.6	13.3	6.9
14–17	92.7	158.4	88.7	236.9
18–24	218.4	725.5	215.4	464.2
25–34	313.0	235.2	317.6	545.4
35–44	323.3	218.9	329.3	716.2
45–64	261.2	129.2	265.4	402.2
65 and over	129.4	278.3	126.7	258.7

Source: U.S. Department of Health, Education, and Welfare, 1977.

TABLE 9.11

Admissions per 100,000 population to State and County Mental Hospitals, by Primary Diagnosis and Ethnicity, 1972

Primary Diagnosis	Total	Hispanic	White	Nonwhite
Total	181.7	133.7	184.3	306.3
Mental	6.0	7.9	5.9	18.9
Alcohol disorders	48.8	20.6	50.3	69.6
Drug disorders	8.6	22.9	7.8	19.3
Organic brain syndromes	12.7	11.3	12.7	22.1
Affective and depressive disorders	24.1	17.4	24.4	12.2
Schizophrenia	50.4	38.4	51.0	118.6
Psychotic disorders (NEC)†	.5	*	.5	5.3
Neurotic disorders (NEC)	2.3	*	2.4	5.1
Personality disorders	13.4	6.2	13.8	23.4
Transient situational disorders and behavior disorders of childhood and adolescence	8.6	*	9.0	4.1
All others	6.5	6.0	6.5	7.8

Source: U.S. Department of Health, Education, and Welfare, 1977.
*Estimates are below acceptable limits of reliability (five cases or fewer).
†NEC = Nowhere Else Classified

errepresented in many of the criminal justice categories, including arrest rates, court trials, sentences, and commitment in penal institutions (Sissons, 1979).

Utilization of Mental Health Services

Practically all of the literature dealing with utilization rates of mental health services by Hispanic Americans indicates that they greatly underutilize the services available. Although the utilization rates are not similar for various Hispanic groups and geographic areas, these rates rarely exceed 50 percent; i.e., Hispanics use services less than one-half the amount that would be expected on the basis of their representation in the general population (President's Commission on Mental Health, 1978). Cuellar (1978) pointed out that this underutilization has been documented in numerous studies over the past twenty years.

Hypotheses have attempted to explain underutilization on various bases, from the potential client to institutional barriers. There seems to be a consensus now, however, that the most important factors are structural in nature and relate primarily to availability, accessibility, and acceptability. Availability means whether or not appropriate services are provided. Accessibility deals with the relative ease of getting to the service. Acceptability is concerned with the psychosocial and sociocultural relevance of the service for the potential recipient. Least attention has been paid to the last factor, which encompasses such variables as language, ethnic sensitivity, and social nuances. Even when services are available and accessible, diagnosis and assessment are likely to be based upon middle-class Anglo values. At the same time, Hispanics are less likely to be prescribed psychotherapy and more likely to receive somatic and psychopharmacological treatment. Similarly, Hispanics are served more often by paraprofessionals than are Anglos (President's Commission on Mental Health, 1978). Another reason suggested for underutilization is that Hispanics rely heavily upon folk medicine experts, or *curanderos*. Although the *curandero* figures prominently in the Hispanic heritage, there are no reliable statistics that document the extent to which folk medicine is used rather than Western medicine.

Underutilization can be reversed, as demonstrated by some creative efforts. One outstanding example is La Frontera, an outpatient facility in Tucson, Arizona, that has been responsive to the needs of Mexican Americans who live within the catchment area. Approximately 40 percent of the target population is Mexican American and 44 percent of the client population at La Frontera are Mexican American. The center uses Mexican American staff and provides a wide range of services to meet the multiple needs of its catchment area population. Traditional modalities are supplemented by a well baby clinic, preschool services, alcoholism services, outreach, and advocacy (Chavez, 1978). Similar programs are offered by the Spanish Hot Line in Washington, D.C.; El Encuentro Spanish Family Guidance Clinic in Miami, Florida; and El Centro de Salud Mental in Oakland, California (Galbis, 1977; Padilla, Ruiz, and Alvarez, 1975).

Status of Mental Health Research

An adequate knowledge base is crucial if there is to be rational planning of mental health services for the Hispanic population. Reliable and valid research data are not available. A review of the literature in 1973, which included approximately five hundred articles, pointed out that a number of serious deficiencies permeated the efforts (Padilla and Ruiz, 1973). The reviewers indicated that research was "plagued by stereotypic interpretations, weak methodological and data-analytic techniques, lack of replicability of findings, and the absence of programmatic research (p. 163)." A review of some two thousand works in 1978 concluded that the quality of the research had not improved (President's Commission on Mental Health, 1978).

Four reasons have been suggested for the poor quality and limitations of the research:

1. Until recently, theories and models in the social and behavioral sci-

ences have been ethnocentric in nature. These constructs have ignored the relevance of sociocultural and linguistic differences between the Anglo and the Hispanic culture.

2. There has been a failure to investigate systematically differences among Hispanic subgroups.
3. There has been a failure to identify and account for the complex interdependence of psychological, sociological, anthropological, and biological factors.
4. There has been a failure to study Hispanics in the context of the microculture within which they exist, namely, twentieth-century American society (President's Commission on Mental Health, 1978).

These indictments make it clear that lack of adequate research and the poor quality of published studies complicate the problems related to the mental health of the Hispanic population. The National Center for Health Statistics has initiated a study that will close the gap in health and nutrition data on Hispanics. The national Hispanic Health and Nutrition Examination Survey (HHANES) should be published early in 1983.

Representation in the Core Mental Health Professions

Hispanic Americans are greatly underrepresented in the core mental health professions of psychiatry, psychology, psychiatric nursing, and social work. This underrepresentation directly affects the utilization of mental health services and the quality of research.

Spanish surnamed psychiatrists accounted for 3.4 percent of the membership of the American Psychiatric Association in 1971 and of this number only 85 (.54 percent) were U.S. residents. In 1976 only 43 Chicanos were in psychiatric residency programs. There were 115 Hispanic psychologists in the United States in 1973, or .5 percent of the total number of 22,500. During the fiscal years 1973–1976 3,213 doctorates were awarded in clinical psychology: 31, or .9 percent, of the recipients were Hispanics. Moreover, the number of Hispanics in Ph.D. programs in clinical psychology in the United States is decreasing.

No specific data on psychiatric nurses are available. Of the approximately one million nurses in the United States, slightly less than one-fifth belong to the American Nurses Association; about one thousand were of Hispanic origin in 1976. In the same year there were twenty-four Hispanic nurses in psychiatric training programs in the United States and Puerto Rico.

Social work has done better numerically, but Hispanics are still underrepresented. Of the forty-three thousand graduates from accredited MSW programs between the years 1969 and 1974, approximately 4 percent were of Hispanic origin. In 1974, Hispanics represented 4.3 percent of the students enrolled in accredited MSW programs (President's Commission on Mental Health, 1978). In 1979, Hispanics accounted for 4.4 percent of full-time students in MSW programs and 4 percent of MSW graduates (Council on Social Work Education, 1975–1979). Hispanic enrollment appears to have leveled off at about 4.5 percent of total enrollment.

The Hispanic panel of the President's Commission on Mental Health (1978) suggested three major reasons for the continuing underrepresentation:

1. the high dropout rate of Hispanics at the elementary and secondary school levels
2. the predominantly disciminatory admission practices, based largely on standardized tests such as the Graduate Record Examination (GRE) and the Medical College Admissions Test (MCAT)
3. the absence of a concerted national effort to recruit and support Hispanic graduate students in the mental health disciplines

There is an urgent need to increase the number of Hispanic professionals in the core mental health professions. Increased numbers would aid in resolving problems of both service delivery and utilization and research. In each of the core mental health disciplines except social work Hispanics represent less than 1 percent of all practitioners, and even in social work representation is below the level that would be expected on the basis of population. Unfortunately, present trends suggest that Hispanics are likely to be grossly underrepresented into the distant future.

Summary

Hispanic Americans are now the second largest minority group in the United States and are projected to be the largest group by the year 2000. Hispanics are slowly being integrated into the mainstream of American society, but they encounter persistent problems in their quest for equality. A team of Hispanic researchers borrowed from Oscar Lewis' concept and labeled this psychosocial situation the culture of poverty (Padilla, Ruiz, and Alvarez, 1975). Factors that combine to create this culture are low income, unemployment, underemployment, undereducation, poor housing, prejudice and discrimination, cultural and linguistic barriers, and powerlessness. As a result, Hispanics are exposed to inordinate life stresses, thus raising their level of mental health risk. In spite of their high-risk status, Hispanics tend to underutilize both inpatient and outpatient mental health services at a rate 50 percent below the level that would be expected on the basis of their representation in the U.S. population. Hispanics are underrepresented in the core mental health professions of social work, psychology, psychiatry, and psychiatric nursing. This underrepresentation is reflected in the unsatisfactory quality of research regarding Hispanic people, as well as in their under-utilization of mental health services.

Native Americans

Obtaining reliable statistics on the number of Native Americans who reside in the United States is a formidable task. The basic reason for this difficulty is that there is no agreed upon definition of who is Native American. Different definitions are used by various federal agencies, and state governments often use other criteria. A few examples demonstrate this definitional maze:

1. anyone with one-quarter or more of Native American blood
2. anyone of Native American descent
3. anyone recognized in the community as Native American
4. residence on a reservation
5. individual's own determination

Census statistics do not clarify the issue: they are often based on other federal records and/or self-reports. According to the 1970 census there were 792,730 Native Americans living in every state of the union and the District of Columbia. This represented a 122 percent increase in population since 1950. Nearly two-thirds lived in eight states (Oklahoma, Arizona, California, New Mexico, Alaska, North Carolina, South Dakota, and Washington). Many people think that the 1970 census grossly undercounted Native Americans. Roughly 25 percent of the Native American population live on reservations; a large percentage of the remainder lives in urban areas and census taking is notoriously inaccurate in urban ghetto areas.

Sociodemographic Characteristics

Native Americans do not consider themselves members of a minority group. According to the President's Commission on Mental Health (1978):

> One of the major problems that faces the American Indians when they deal with government is the imposition of the status of minority persons. While the Indian is a minority person in the sense that he or she is a person of color, the only commonality the Indian shares with other minorities is that of racism and poverty. (P. 956)

Within the federal system, the government's relationship with the Native American people is regulated by solemn treaties and by layers of judicial and legislative actions (President's Commission on Mental Health, 1978).

The various tribes perceive themselves as sovereign nations but see their sovereignty as having been vitiated by federal policies that have rendered tribal governments powerless and attempted to assimilate reservation residents into the mainstream of Anglo culture. These efforts have made the Native American a "captive within a free society" (President's Commission on Mental Health, 1978) and encouraged migration from the reservations to urban centers.

In 1930, only 10 percent of Native Americans lived in urban areas; by 1970, this figure had climbed to 45 percent. Nevertheless, Native Americans remain the most rural group in America. The shift to urban life is particularly apparent among males and females aged twenty to forty. Seven standard metropolitan statistical areas have ten thousand or more Native Americans living within their confines: Los Angeles, Oklahoma City, New York City, Phoenix, Minneapolis–St. Paul, San Francisco–Oakland, and Tulsa. About half of the urban Native Americans live in poverty neighborhoods in the inner city. (Native Americans seem to prefer Asian or Mexican American and white neighborhoods; however, in New York City they are concentrated in the black slums of Brooklyn.)

The urban migration of young and middle-aged adults has created an urban-rural dichotomy that is apparent in several indices, such as employment, educational level, and adequacy of housing. For example, employment opportunities appear to be better for Native Americans in urban areas than in rural areas for both males and females. Employment-unemployment statistics include only those individuals who are either working or seeking employment but do not give information on labor force participation; however, many job seekers eventually resign from the labor force after meeting with repeated failure. The labor force participation rates of urban Native American men (72 percent) and women (42 percent) are near the national levels of 77 percent for men and 41 percent for women. In contrast, rates for rural Native American men (56 percent) and women (29 percent) are far lower than those of any other group in our society. Jobs held by urban Native Americans suggest upward mobility: 23 percent of males are in skilled blue-collar jobs, 48 percent of females are in white-collar occupations, 12 percent of females are professional workers, and 29 percent of females are clerical workers (U.S. Department of Health, Education, and Welfare, 1974).

Income, of course, is closely related to employment. Native Americans have the lowest individual income of any group in America. In every income category, Native Americans earn less than persons in the remainder of the U.S. population. Of all Native American males 55 percent have incomes of less than $4,000 per year, in contrast to approximately 30 percent of men in the total U.S. population. Among rural Native American men almost 64 percent earn less than $4,000 per year. Overall, Native Americans have the lowest median income of any group in the United States but at the same time they have among the largest families. Table 9.12 indicates 1970 income levels of individuals and families by sex and place of residence.

Poverty is also reflected in housing conditions (Table 9.13). In general, Native Americans have trouble finding adequate housing because they encounter discriminatory practices, have large families, and lack information regarding housing alternatives. Urban Native Americans are fourteen times more likely than the total U.S. urban population to live in households without toilets. In rural areas, almost half of all Native American dwellings are without toilets. Approximately two-thirds of all rural Native Americans do not have water in their houses. This proportion is eight times greater than that for in the total U.S. population.

The educational level of Native Americans as a group is improving, but more so for urban families (Table 9.14). Of this group, 26 percent have had eight years of education or less, equal to the level in the total U.S. population. In 1960, 28 percent of urban Native Americans were high school graduates and by 1970 this figure had risen to 42 percent. In contrast, 48 percent of rural Native Americans have not gone beyond elementary school and only 23 percent are high school graduates. The school attendance of

TABLE 9.12
Income Profile of Native Americans, 1970

Income of Persons 16 and Over	U.S. Total	Total Native American	Urban Native American	Rural Native American
Under $4,000				
Male	31%	55%	46%	64%
Female	68%	80%	74%	86%
$10,000 and over				
Male	25.2%	8.5%	12.5%	4.7%
Female	3.2%	1.5%	2.1%	0.8%
Median				
Male	$6,614	$3,509	$4,568	$2,749
Female	2,404	1,697	2,023	1,356
Income of families				
Under $4,000	15%	34%	24%	44%
$10,000 and over	47%	22%	31%	15%
Median	$9,590	$5,832	$7,323	$4,649
Income of families with female heads				
Under $4,000	41%	61%	55%	68%
$10,000 and over	18%	6.4%	8.4%	4.3%
Median	$4,962	$3,198	$3,932	$2,704

Source: U.S. Department of Health, Education, and Welfare, 1974.

TABLE 9.13
Housing and Sanitation Data for Native Americans, 1974

	Urban		Rural	
	U.S. Total	Native Americans	U.S. Total	Native Americans
Persons per room				
1.00 or less	92.5%	81.3%	89.9%	55.0%
1.01–1.50	5.7	12.2	7.1	15.4
1.51 or more				
(severe crowding)	1.9	6.4	3.0	28.6
Sanitation facilities				
No water	.3%	.9%	8.7%	67.4%
No toilet	.6	8.6	13.6	48.0

Source: U.S. Department of Health, Education, and Welfare, 1974.

urban and rural Native Americans aged fourteen to seventeen is practically the same, 86 percent and 87 percent, respectively.

Language is a related problem in discrimination and education that has not been addressed adequately for Native Americans. Approximately 35 percent of this population have a Native American language as their mother tongue. As with the Hispanic population, language poses educational barriers and affects the entire psychosocial-cultural spectrum.

The state of Native American health is deplorable but is improving in some disease categories. However, morbidity and mortality rates must be evaluated against the birth rate, which is nearly twice as high among Native Americans as among the U.S. population in general.

Native Americans show death rates at early ages in excess of national averages. Deaths among Native Americans less than one year old constitute 10 percent of deaths in this group, compared to 4 percent for the total U.S. population. Similar proportions are found in the preschool years. There is a particularly high mortality rate between the ages of five and twenty-four. Especially high are the death rates for accidents, cirrhosis of the liver, influenza and pneumonia, and diabetes mellitus. Simply stated, Native Americans are more likely to die at a faster rate than are other persons in the U.S. population (Table 9.15). For example, Table 9.15 indicates that the death rate among Native Americans is approximately one-third higher than that for the U.S. white population.

Mental Health Risk

Social, economic, and housing conditions all affect mental health. As a group, Native Americans live under conditions that make them particularly

TABLE 9.14
Schooling Completed by Native Americans, by Age and Sex, 1970

Years of Schooling and Age	Males Native Americans			Females Native Americans		
	U.S.	Urban	Rural	U.S.	Urban	Rural
8 years of school or less						
16–24	11.0	12.0	23.0	8.0	11.0	19.0
25–34	11.0	17.0		10.0	17.0	34.0
35–44	19.0	29.0	52.0	15.0	26.0	48.0
45–64	33.0	40.0	63.0	30.0	36.0	60.0
65 and over	61.0	69.0	84.0	55.0	61.0	81.0
High school graduate						
16–24	66.0	48.0	26.0	71.0	48.0	30.0
25–34	72.0	58.0	39.0	71.0	53.0	36.0
35–44	61.0	45.0	25.0	63.0	46.0	24.0
45–64	46.0	37.0	19.0	49.0	38.0	19.0
4 years of college or more						
16–24	6.5	1.9	.1	6.1	1.4	.4
25–34	19.0	8.9	3.0	12.1	5.8	1.9
35–44	17.5	7.8	2.4	8.9	5.0	1.2
45–64	10.8	5.6	2.0	7.1	4.1	1.7
65 and over	6.3	4.1	.6	4.9	3.7	1.1

Source: Task Force Eight. "Report on Urban and Rural Non-reservation Indians," *Final Report to the American Indian Policy Review Committee.* Washington, D.C.: U.S. Government Printing Office, 1976.

The high accident rate is closely correlated to use of alcohol.

Broken families, divorce, juvenile delinquency, illegitimacy, child neglect and abuse have become common in a population where they had rarely existed before. (Task Force Six. "Report on Indian Health," *Final Report to the American Indian Policy Review Committee.* Washington, D.C.: U.S. Government Printing Office, 1976, p. 15.)

Alcoholism and related factors, homicide, suicide, and family disorders are major mental health problems. Among the Native American population, almost 50 percent of suicide attempts are alcohol related. Alcoholism is the primary mental health problem among Native Americans. This condition plays a role in family breakdown, criminal activity, job instability, and a host of other social, economic, political, and spiritual problems.

The high level of mental health risk must be evaluated within the context of the history of Native Americans and their association with the U.S. government:

Indians have lost their lands and their economic base, and their culture has been seriously undermined. They have been taught that they are inferior and that their most precious values were false. Epidemics and other upheavals have disrupted family and community systems. Aggravating these conditions are almost two centuries of autocratic, uncoordinated federal control, substandard living conditions, insufficient diets, poor physical health, meager employment opportunities, and inappropriate education.

But perhaps the principal reason for the emotional distress of many Indians is the gap between their culture and the dominant white culture, and the strain of fruitless past efforts to close the gap. (Task Force Six. "Report on Indian Health," *Final Report to the American Indian Policy Review Committee.* Washington, D.C.: U.S. Government Printing Office, 1976, p. 68.)

Thus, Native Americans historically have experienced dependence, hopelessness, and powerlessness. Memmi (1965) referred to the parties in such a situation as the colonizer and the colonized, with the Native American the colonized here and the American government the colonizer. Successful adjustment on the part of the Native American often has meant how well he had incorporated the values of mainstream U.S. culture and rejected his indigenous culture. Indeed, there has been an organized effort to get the Native American to leave the reservation and to become assimilated into the dominant Anglo culture.

Native Americans have been denied the right to control their own destiny. Policymakers in government have developed and implemented plans designed to foster dependence in a people who historically were proud and self-sufficient:

The view of American History from the Native American side of the frontier offers a curiously reversed image of the rise and fall of nations. Commonly, historians of the U.S. describe the period of 1607 to 1776 as the "colonial period," for most Indian tribes this same stretch of years represents a period of relative independence and equality between red nations and white colonies. . . . America's rise to world power entailed the reduction of the Native American to the status of a captive population, euphemistically termed wards. (President's Commission on Mental Health, 1978, p. 958.)

Utilization of Mental Health Services

The utilization of mental health services by any ethnic group is correlated closely with availability, accessibility, and acceptability. Considerable data suggest that mental health service delivery to Native American populations is a failure on each of these three variables. Some distinction, however, needs to be made between services provided through community mental health centers and those provided through the Indian Health Service on reservations. Community mental health centers are supposed to be the primary mental health agency for most segments of the population; however, this does not hold true for Native Americans. The President's Commission on Mental Health (1978) documented the nonavailability, nonaccessibility, and nonacceptability of services in community mental health centers.

The current policy of the federal government is self-determination for Native Americans, yet in the mental health field these people are denied the right to design their own programs and centers, to apply for funds, or to participate in ongoing community mental health center programs:

There is a paucity of data about Community Mental Health Center services to the Indian population. While some centers utilize various statistics, many Indian people feel that statistics are not reliable and cannot tell of many rejections and barriers to service. There is not one Community Mental Health Center on an Indian reservation. (President's Commission on Mental Health, 1978, p. 988.)

Mental health services are offered on reservations through eight regional health centers operated by the Indian Health Service. The mental health programs and the Indian Health Service are funded separately and have independent chains of command. Each of the area mental health offices provides only limited services because of staffing and budgetary shortages. A comprehensive needs assessment has never been done and as a result services are fragmented and randomly delivered. Hospital care is not available in six of the eight areas and the existing physical facilities are inadequate. Contract hospitalization is used as an alternative, but it removes the patient from his familial support system and Native American consumers feel that they are not welcome in outside facilities because of prejudice and/or cultural barriers. Psychiatric intervention for patients who require acute services is critically limited, in part because of the shortage of mental health professionals. Paraprofessionals assume a large portion of the workload for direct intervention, as well as for collateral contact and tangible services. Some alcoholism treatment programs have been managed by Native Americans, but most programs are staffed by Anglos. A few model or demonstration projects have been developed, such as the suicide prevention program in Portland, Oregon.

There is some push to utilize the special skills of traditional Native American healers as an adjunct to therapy or as the treatment of choice. It is argued that the "medicine men excel in the prevention and treatment of mental and psychosomatic illnesses." The National Institute of Mental Health established a training program for medicine men in the late 1960s so that they could provide treatment and teaching services in the community. Even though the combination of traditional and Western medicine is controversial, it may prove an effective treatment tool (Task Force Six, Final Report to the American Indian Policy Review Committee, 1977).

Status of Mental Health Research

Padilla and Ruiz (1973, p. 163) pointed out that research on Hispanics has been "plagued by stereotypic interpretations, weak methodological and data-analytic techniques, lack of replicability of findings, and the absence of programmatic research." The same arguments apply to research on the Native American, but with an additional aspect. Much of this research seems to have been structured to elicit negative data and to depict the subject in an unfavorable light. Empirical reports emphasize severe poverty, major health problems, inadequate educational resources and opportunities, and the perpetual dependence created by federal government policy. A recent report concluded that "probably no other group in the U.S. has been more studied and reported on, billions of dollars have been spent . . . in the name of the Indian people. All of these reports have had little impact on improving the quality of life for Indian people (President's Commission on Mental Health, 1978, p. 960).

Native Americans themselves have begun to reject study proposals by non–Native American researchers. Issues regarding content, methodology, and interpretation of findings are being reviewed by Native Americans and approval of the tribe is required before a study can be started (Trimble, 1977). There is the possibility of distortion from the point of problem formulation through question formulation, data analysis, and data interpretation. Even the presence of a non–Native American on the reservation doing research adds an artifact (Trimble, 1977). Trimble reviewed personality research among Native Americans and concluded that the results did not provide a base for program development or problem-solving; the findings usually were placed within non–Native American theoretical frameworks; and the methodology and procedures approached research questions from perspectives foreign to respondents, which tended to restrict elaboration from the Native American view. In essence, "research tends to be ethnocentric, narrow in focus, and full of misinterpretations" (Trimble, 1977, p. 162).

Sufficient reliable data are not available to make the kinds of decisions that are needed to develop effective mental health programs. Research should be sensitive to tribal and geographic differences. For example, the living situation of urban and rural Native Americans is very different. Similarly, Alaskan tribespeople differ in important ways from Native Americans living in the rural Southwest.

Representation in the Core Mental Health Professions

Native American representation in the core mental health professions is virtually nonexistent. According to the Association of American Indian Physicians there are only ninety-six physicians of one-eighth degree or more of Native American blood; there are only thirteen psychiatrists, and it is not clear whether these are included in the total of ninety-six (President's Commission on Mental Health, 1978). There are only two Native American psychiatric nurses, and only eleven Native Americans have a master's degree in psychology (President's Commission on Mental Health, 1978).

Social workers have a slightly better representation, but the totals continue to be dismal. By 1976, 173 Native Americans had secured an MSW. In 1977, there were approximately 55 MSW candidates and this number remained the same in 1979 (Council on Social Work Education, 1975–1979). About 25 Native Americans have earned a doctoral degree in social work.

Much of the training in mental health has been concentrated at the paraprofessional level. For example, only one program in the United States is dedicated to graduating Native American physicians and this is at the University of North Dakota. Paraprofessional training is valuable in that it prepares indigenous people to provide mental health services; at the same time, however, it limits the quality of services delivered. This deficiency, however, must be balanced against the delivery of mental health services by non–Native American personnel, who may be culturally insensitive. The need for cultural sensitivity was pointed out strikingly by Goodtracks (1973). One of the recommendations of the Native American subpanel of the President's Commission on Mental Health (1978) was that support be given to programs to train Native Americans in the mental health professions. At the current rate of increase of representation in the core mental health professions, the Indians are losing another battle to the white man.

Summary

In relationship to the other groups included in this chapter, the Native American population is the smallest, numbering about 800,000 persons. It is, however, probably the most mobile group: in 1930 only 10 percent of Native Americans were urban dwellers, but by 1970 over 45 percent resided in metropolitan areas. The rapidity of this shift is dramatized when it is recognized that the Native American urban population doubled in the decade 1960–1970. Additionally, this migration has been effected primarily by young and middle-aged people. A rural-urban dichotomy has developed as a result of this mobility. Native Americans residing in rural areas score near the bottom of the socio-economic ladder on practically every index of affluence. Native Americans have the lowest income of any group in America; in 1974 46 percent of urban Native Americans earned less than $4,000, while 64 percent of their rural counterparts had earnings at this level.

The health status of Native Americans is also remarkable. Morbidity and mortality rates are especially high. Accidents, cirrhosis of the liver, influenza and pneumonia, diabetes mellitus, suicide, and homicide are major causes of death. Alcoholism is the foremost health problem. In spite of the high level of mental health risk, Native Americans underutilize mental health services, primarily because of problems of availability, accessibility, and acceptability. Language is also a problem: 35 percent of all Native Americans speak an indigenous American language as their mother tongue.

In short, Native Americans face problems similar to those of other special population groups.

Issues, Problems, and Prospects

The mental health status of Native Americans, blacks, and Hispanics highlights their marginal existence in U.S. society. Such marginality greatly affects mental health. Assessing the level of mental health functioning is difficult because of contradictory research findings. Three factors make investigation problematic: there is a lack of agreement among researchers as to what is mental health or mental illness; many existing epidemiological studies have serious methodological and analytical problems; and many of these studies have relied upon simplistic analytical procedures such as frequencies and percentages rather than on multivariate analysis (President's Commission on Mental Health, 1978; Warheit et al., 1975; Willie et al., 1975). Although a comparative research paradigm, in which various ethnic groups are compared with whites, has some utility, there is a need for research designs that examine objectively mental health functioning in diverse subgroups within specified communities.

A much debated issue is whether members of one ethnic group can provide mental health services effectively to members of another ethnic group. This question has not been answered to date and is not likely to be answered conclusively in the immediate future. There is some agreement, however, regarding variables that appear to be correlated with utilization rates. The attitude of the provider can encourage or discourage continuance by the service seeker. Understanding on the part of the provider of the social problems, such as racism and poverty, faced by the service seeker is crucial. Knowledge of the culture and language of the consumer of services by the provider also seems to be correlated directly with service utilization.

Each of the three population groups studied in this chapter is underrepresented in the core mental health professions. Adequate representation would help resolve utilization problems, but in addition these professionals could aid in assessing the effects of racism and second-class citizenship upon the mental health of their communities. Representation at policymaking and decisionmaking levels could influence resource distribution, research planning, and service delivery. Members of ethnic groups are already beginning to insist upon a more equitable distribution of resources. Similarly, there is insistence that ethnic group members be involved in every stage of research directed at their group.

Native Americans, blacks, and Hispanics are at-risk populations. A mixture of assertiveness by members of these three groups, enlightenment and belief in equity on the part of some Anglos, and slight policy shifts at federal, state, and local levels has brought about minimal changes. But the goal of mental health for all Americans is still one to be attained.

The environmental, economic, and cultural problems and the powerlessness in black, Native American, and Hispanic communities represent only a few of the many societal factors that cause acute stress for these Americans. Changing the societal context in which these populations live is clearly beyond the province of mental health providers. Advocacy within the mental health field can, however, lead the way toward improving the quality of the social milieu and insuring the survival and growth of our social order. In addition, effective advocacy can help to reorient mental health services. A review of the mental health literature reveals that until recently there has been little real concern for blacks, Hispanics, and Native Americans. This has been manifested in stereotypes regarding character structure, differential diagnostic patterns, discrimination in services provided, and, most important, overemphasis upon emotional and psychological explanations for mental illness (Cannon and Locke, 1977; Mayfield, 1972; Shannon, 1973).

Any analysis of the mental health status of blacks, Native Americans, and Hispanics that ignores, minimizes, or negates the degree to which racism affects the atmosphere in which they develop is, at best, ludicrous. The mental health status of ethnic groups must be assessed within the framework of their culture and community, as well as their community's relationship to the larger society. This task is not amenable to an analysis based on white middle-class culture and values. Indeed, viewed more objectively, many aspects of ethnic behavior may not be pathological but appropriate and constructive (Jones, 1979).

REFERENCES

BALAH, P. "A Racial Comparison of the Admission, Diagnosis, and Release of Patients in the State Mental Hospitals of Florida." Master's thesis, Florida State University, 1970.

BESTMAN, E. W. "Delivery of Mental Health Services to Black Americans." Paper prepared for the President's Commission on Mental Health, 1978.

BILLINGSLEY, A. *Black Families in White America*. Englewood Cliffs: Prentice-Hall, 1968.

CANNON, M. S., and LOCKE, B. A. "Being Black Is Detrimental to One's Mental Health: Myth or Reality." *Phylon* 1977, *38*(4): 408–428.

CARKHUFF, R., and PIERCE, R. "Differential Effects of the Therapist's Race and Social Class upon Patient Depth of Self-exploration in the Clinical Interview." *Journal of Consulting Psychlogy* 1967, *31*(6):632–634.

CHAVEZ, N. "The Issues of Non-responsiveness vs. Responsive Mental Health Services for Mexican-Americans: Implications for Practice." In Federico Soufleé and Joan Valdez (eds.), *Proceedings of Texas–New Mexico Symposium on the Delivery of Mental Health Services to Mexican-Americans,* vol. 1. Houston: 1978.

COLE, O. J. "Research Issues: Projected Way of Dealing with Future Mental Health Needs of the Nation." Paper prepared for the President's Commission on Mental Health, 1977.

Council on Social Work Education. *Statistics on Social Work Education in the United States.* New York: Council on Social Work Education, 1975–1977, 1979.

CUELLAR, I. "Underutilization of Mental Health Facilities and Services by Mexican-Americans: Who, Where, How Much, and Why." In Federico Soufleé and Joan Valdez (eds.), *Proceedings of the Texas–New Mexico Symposium on the Delivery of Mental Health Services to Mexican-Americans,* vol. 1. Houston: 1978.

DOHRENWEND, B. P., and DOHRENWEND, B. S. *Social Status and Psychological Disorder.* New York: Wiley, 1969.

Fried, M. "Social Differences in Mental Health." In J. Kosa, A. Antonovsky, and I. Zola (eds.), *Poverty and Health.* New York: Commonwealth Fund, 1969.

FISHER, J. "Negroes and Whites and Rates of Mental Illness: Reconsideration of a Myth." *Psychiatry* 1969, *32*(4):428–446.

FUNNYE, C. "The Militant Black Social Worker and the Urban Hustle." *Social Work* 1970, *15*(2):5–12.

GABLIS, R. "Mental Health in a Hispano Community." *Urban Health* 1977, *6*(6): 31–35.

GARDNER, W. "The Differential Effects of Race, Education, and Experience in Helping." *Journal of Clinical Psychology* 1972, *28*(1):87–89.

GARY, L. E. "Mental Health Research in the Black Community." In E. Cash, L.

E. Gary, L. R. Mathis, and T. Thompson (eds.), *Key Mental Health Issues in the Black Community*. Washington, D.C.: Institute for Urban Affairs and Research, Howard University, 1974.

GOODTRACKS, J. G. "Native American Noninterference." *Social Work* 1973, *18*(6):30–34.

GORWITZ, K. "The Mental Health of the Negro." *Maryland Department of Mental Hygiene Statistical Newsletter,* February 10, 1966, Pp. 4–9.

GRIER, W. H., and COBBS, P. M. *Black Rage.* New York: Basic Books, 1968.

HARE, B. R. "Racism and the Mental Health of Black Americans: The Societal Level." Paper prepared for the President's Commission on Mental Health, 1978.

HARRISON, D. K. "Race as a Counselor-Client Variable in Counseling and Psychotherapy: A Review of the Research." *Counseling Psychologist* 1975, *5*(2):124–133.

JONES, D. L. "African-American Clients: Clinical Practice Issues." *Social Work* 1979, *24*(2):112–118.

JONES, E. "Social Class and Psychotherapy: A Critical Review of Research." *Psychiatry* 1974, *37*(4):307–320.

JONES, M. H., and JONES, M. C. "The Neglected Client." *Black Scholar* 1970, *1*(1):35–42.

KARNO, N., and EDGERTON, R. B. "Perceptions of Mental Illness in a Mexican-American Community." *Archives of General Psychiatry* 1969, *20*(2):233–238.

LEWIS, H. *Child Rearing among Low Income Families.* Washington, D.C.: Health and Welfare Council of the National Capital Area, 1961.

LORION, R. P. "Mental Health and the Disadvantaged." in H. Rubenstein, and M. H. Bloch (eds.), *Things That Matter: Influences on Helping Relationships.* New York: Macmillan, 1982.

MACIAS, R. F. "U. S. Hispanics in 2000 A.D.: Projecting the Number." *Agenda* 1977, *7*( ):16–20.

MAYFIELD, W. C. "Mental Health in the Black Community." *Social Work* 1972, *17* 106–110.

MEMMI, A. *The Colonizer and the Colonized.* Boston: Beacon, 1965.

MILLER, K. S., and JOEL, J. "Mental Health." In K. S. Miller and R. M. Dreger (eds.), *Comparative Studies of Blacks and Whites in the U.S.* New York: Seminar, 1973.

MIZIO, E. "White Worker–Minority Client." *Social Work* 1972, *17*(3):82–86.

MOYNIHAN, D. P. *The Negro Family: The Case for National Action.* Washington, D.C.: Department of Labor, 1965.

NOBLES, W. W. "The Right of Culture: A Declaration for the Provision of Culturally Sensitive Mental Health Services and the Issue of Protected Status." In *Multi-cultural Issues in Mental Health Services: Strategies toward Equity.* Sacramento: California Health and Welfare Agency, 1979.

OZAWA, M. N. "Social Welfare: The Minority Share." *Social Work* 1972, *17*(3):33.

PADILLA, A. M., and RUIZ, R. A. *Latino Mental Health: A Review of Literature.* DHEW pub. no. (HSM) 73–9143. Washington, D.C.: U.S. Government Printing Office, 1973.

PADILLA, A. M., RUIZ, R. A., and ALVAREZ, R. "Community Mental Health Services for the Spanish Speaking/Surnamed Population." *American Psychologist* 1975, *30*(9):892–905.

President's Commission on Mental Health. *Report to the President,* vol. 3. Washington, D.C.: U.S. Government Printing Office, 1978.

RAINWATER, L. "Some Aspects of Lower Class Sexual Behavior." *Journal of Social Issues* 1966, *22*(2):96–108.

RUDOR, M. H., and SANTANGELO, N. *Health Status of Minorities and Low Income Groups.* Washington, D.C.: Public Health Service–Health Resource Administration, 1978.

SHANNON, B. E. "The Impact of Racism on Personality Development." *Social Casework* 1973, *74*(9):519–525.

SISSONS, P. L. *The Hispanic Experience of Criminal Justice.* New York: Hispanic Research Center, Fordham University, 1979.

SMITH, W. D., BURLEN, A. K., MOSELY, N. H., and WHITNEY, W. M. *Minority Issues in Mental Health.* Reading, Mass.: Addison-Wesley, 1978.

SUE, D. W., and SUE, D. "Barriers to Cross-cultural Counseling." *Journal of Counseling Psychology* 1977, *24*(5):420–429.

Task Force Eight, *Final Report to the American Indian Policy Review Committee* "Report on Urban and Rural Non-reservation Indians". Washington, D.C.: U.S. Government Printing Office, 1976.

Task Force Eleven, *Final Report to the American Indian Policy Review Committee* "Report on Alcohol and Drug Abuse". Washington, D.C.: U.S. Government Printing Office, 1976.

Task Force Six, *Final Report to the American Indian Policy Review Committee* "Report on Indian Health". Washington, D.C.: U.S. Government Printing Office, 1976.

THOMAS, A., and SILLEN, S. *Racism and Psychiatry.* New York: Brunner/Mazel, 1972.

TRIMBLE, J. E. "The Sojourner in the American Indian Community: Methodological Issues and Concerns." *Journal of Social Issues* 1977, *33*(4):159–174.

U.S. Bureau of the Census. *1970 Census of Population Supplementary Reports: Persons of Spanish Ancestry.* Washington, D.C.: U.S. Government Printing Office, 1973.

———. *Current Population Reports: Persons of Spanish Origin in the United States, March 1975.* Washington, D.C.: U.S. Government Printing Office, 1976.

———. *Current Population Reports: Persons of Spanish Origin in the United States, March 1978.* Washington, D.C.: U.S. Government Printing Office, 1979.(a)

———. *The Social and Economic Status of the Black Population in the United States: An Historical View, 1970–1978.* Washington, D.C.: U.S. Government Printing Office, 1979.(b)

U.S. Bureau of the Census. "United States Summary." *1980 Census of Population and Housing: Advance Report.* Washington, D.C.: U.S. Government Printing Office, 1981.

U.S. Department of Health, Education, and Welfare. *A Study of Selected Socioeconomic Characteristics of Ethnic Minorities Based on the 1970 Census.* vol. 3: *American Indians.* Washington, D.C.: U.S. Government Printing Office, 1974.

———. *Health of the Disadvantaged Chart Book, 1977.* DHEW pub. no. (HRA) 77–628. Washington, D.C.: U.S. Government Printing Office, 1977.

Urban Research Review 1980, *6*(1).

WARHEIT, G. R., HOLYER, C. E., and AREY, S. A. "Race and Mental Illness: An Epidemiological Update." *Journal of Health and Social Behavior* 1976, *15*(3):243–256.

WILLIE, C., KRAMER, B. M., and BROWN, S. (eds.). *Racism and Mental Health.* Pittsburgh: University of Pittsburgh Press, 1973.

CHAPTER 10

Interdisciplinary Teams

James W. Callicutt
Pedro J. Lecca

CHAPTER 3 INDICATED that psychiatric social work began in hospitals and clinics and enjoyed a close relationship with medicine from the outset. With the development of the child guidance clinic, the team of psychiatrist, psychologist, and social worker became the rule; neurologists and pediatricians also participated in interdisciplinary treatment efforts.

In contemporary mental health settings, where acute and chronic mental health problems are addressed, the need for diverse professional and technical skills is indisputable. Indeed, the multiple functions of a state hospital, Veterans Administration neuropsychiatric hospital, child guidance clinic, or community mental health center make it impossible for the mission of the institution to be accomplished by a single occupational group. Just as schools need the services of teachers, librarians, guidance counselors, nutritionists, maintenance workers, and office staff, so mental health institutions require the services of a variety of personnel, including psychiatrists, psychologists, social workers, nurses, secretarial staff, custodians, and, for facilities providing residential care, dietitians and other specialists.

The basic interdisciplinary mental health team in the 1980s represents psychiatry, psychology, social work, and mental health nursing. Membership on these teams may be expanded considerably beyond the core disciplines, depending on the setting, to include vocational rehabilitation specialists, occupational therapists, counseling psychologists, and others.

Looking at organizational arrangements, Pusić (1974) distinguished four types of cooperating systems. He identified the team network as the most complex of these types. "This highly complex structure is composed of people as specialists (as sources of information) who are combined into teams on the basis of equality among members" (pp. 193–194).

New (1968) examined the concept of teamwork from an analytic perspective. Using six assumptions in teamwork he developed a paradigm that may be applied in explaining success or failure in teamwork. His paradigm of cognitive dissonance used teamwork assumptions involved in the concepts of (1) equality, (2) knowledge, (3) professions, (4) marginality, (5) task, and (6) domain. He analyzed these assumptions of teamwork along the axes of functional rationality and substantive rationality. Functional rationality refers to the need to "get something done" whereas substantive rationality acts on the thought by the individual which reveals intellect and insight. New pointed out that incongruities in action occur when there is a difference between functional rationality and substantive rationality. Application of New's paradigm in specific situations reveals that the assumptions of teamwork do not always stand. He noted, for example, that equality, as an assumption, may not hold up under certain circumstances; that is, all members of the team may indeed *not* be perceived and treated as co-equal members. Thus, the use of New's paradigm may contribute to a better understanding of teamwork by viewing it through the lens of commonly held assumptions in specific circumstances.

However, we can be sure that the quality of mental health care will depend ultimately on the knowledge, skills, and sensitivity of those team members providing this care. Perhaps only through an interdisciplinary team approach can comprehensive delivery systems containing those elements that foster quality mental health care be achieved.

The task is formidable. For example, according to the 1975 special census (U.S. Bureau of the Census, 1975), a large percentage of ethnic minorities did not have appropriate or accessible services, even though social, economic, and environmental factors render these populations particularly vulnerable to acute and prolonged psychological and emotional distress (see Chapter 9). Adolescents also are at risk, suffering from fast social change and conflicting social values. Their vulnerability is underscored by federal reports of a high suicide rate for adolescents (Chilman, 1979). The aged likewise are not receiving adequate mental health care, even though mental illness and emotional distress are prevalent in this population. The President's Commission on Mental Health (1978) estimated that some 25 percent of the population suffer from mild to moderate depression, anxiety, and other emotional disorders at any given time. To meet these needs requires improved coordination of mental health services with general health and other human services, along with an interdisciplinary approach to the delivery of mental health services.

Advantages and Problems

As mentioned previously, mental health settings confront complex problems that a single discipline cannot solve. The interdisciplinary effort required to meet the client population's diverse needs must proceed on the basis of cooperation, collaboration, and reciprocity. Clearly, the development of an interdisciplinary team may not always be easy. For example, new members of the team may become victims of a group ritual of exclusion (Bickford, 1974). "Poor team dynamics [may result] from conflicts among disciplines, personal frictions, defense of professional territory, or domination by one discipline or team member" (Chamberlin, 1980, p. 439).

Despite the difficulty of assembling and running a mental health team, the team approach has a number of advantages. The advantages or costs to clients should be the primary consideration.

Callicutt (1971), described the work of a team on a psychiatric ward. The team included a psychologist (the ward administrator), clinical social worker, psychiatric nurse, nursing assistants, secretary, and clothing clerk. This team established the practice of keeping an agenda book, and any member of the ward staff could put an item on the agenda by entering it in the book. Staff on all shifts were encouraged to enumerate their concerns and questions regarding individual patients, as well as policy. Then, on each weekday morning the staff would confer; once the twenty-four-hour nursing report had been reviewed, the ward agenda book would be considered. While participation by the secretary and clothing clerk was not required, the clinical staff participated regularly. Usually the psychologist (ward administrator) chaired the conference, but the chair went to other members of the staff on an informal rotation when the psychologist was not present.

There was a clear expectation that each member would be responsible for presenting his or her position on any item that was discussed. Most matters were agreed upon through informal discussion. However, if there were disagreements, staff members were encouraged forcefully to present their views. Then a vote was taken, with the team agreeing to support the majority decision. This procedure helped bring a consistent response from each member of the staff with regard to issues concerning individual patients and ward policy and governance.

Advantages to the patients of a consistent approach were apparent. In instances of disagreement, patients were candidly told that the staff had to abide by the team decision even though some members of the staff may have opposed the decision. This approach created an atmosphere of security and trust. (See also Brill, 1976; Hirschowitz, 1973; Johnson, Crocket, Freehlich, and Messick, 1975; Schwartz, 1974; Shapiro and Gudeman, 1974; Stanton and Schwartz, 1954).

The team approach is also desirable in traditional and nontraditional mental health settings because collaboration among professionals contributes to sound decisionmaking. This advantage to patients is important to practitioners in an era of substantial malpractice litigation.

Training

Smith (1974) identified the benefits of interdisciplinary training:

1. enhancing the professionals' capacity to work together "efficiently, harmoniously, and knowledgeably"
2. teaching more fruitfully the overlapping knowledge and skills through interdisciplinary class and field learning vehicles
3. facilitating student and faculty learning from and about one another through carefully planned mixes of students and faculty
4. increasing the efficiency of teaching about the specialized area of community mental health
5. identifying differences among the professions
6. enhancing professional identity through emphasizing the uniqueness of each profession

He suggested that curriculums include theory and skills bearing upon the family and family intervention; child mental health; the community, including community dynamics and organization; social policy, and planning.

Smith (1974) also enumerated the obstacles, both organizational and attitudinal, to the implementation of interdisciplinary training programs. Organizational obstacles, for example, relate to organization by, and emphasis on, disciplines; whereas attitudinal obstacles include concern over the loss of professional identity. The division of universities into academic departments and professional schools is another organizational barrier to the implementation of interdisciplinary training programs.

Spensley and Langsley (1977) described a one-year interdisciplinary training program for first-year psychiatric residents, psychology interns, and master's level students in social work and mental health nursing: "Task analysis suggests that such training should develop knowledge and skill in diagnosis-assessment, treatment, consultation, research, teaching, prevention, and professional identity. . . . a mental health team can provide economical, effective, and comprehensive services to a population" (p. 75).

While not under the rubric of training, evaluation of the interdisciplinary team is a related issue raised by the contemporary emphasis upon accountability. Folkins and Spensley (1977) discussed the implementation of a growth oriented peer rating system "devised in response to a request from members of a community mental health team for a positive method of self-evaluation" (p. 331). Exceptional opportunities for the development of an esprit de corps are available through the vehicle of a mental health team.

Nontraditional Settings

For an interdisciplinary team approach to succeed in nontraditional mental health settings, verbal communications about cases must be supplemented by formal and informal written reports and memos.

Experience has shown that the team approach in nontraditional mental health settings such as schools, nursing homes, and general hospitals is as effective as the approach in traditional mental health settings. Benedetto (1977) described a California program in a general hospital that provided mental health patients with an alternative to hospital confinement and the opportunity to resolve emotional crises in less than a day. The program emphasized crisis intervention, family therapy, chemotherapy, and immediate referral follow-up. This program was staffed by a psychiatrist, a psychologist, and a social worker, as well as two psychiatric nurses and three mental health technicians.

Other nontraditional mental health settings have used interdisciplinary teams. Greiff (1978) looked at the historical development of occupational mental health and the ways in which industrial psychiatrists have integrated contributions from medicine, clinical psychiatry, psychology, social work, and education to enhance the personality adjustment and productivity of workers. Sherr and Goffi (1977) described a long-term study involving a 152-bed geriatric home and a psychiatric social work team. The team approach resulted in significantly improved life satisfaction among the residents. Burchill (1977) discussed a geriatric treatment facility that used an interdisciplinary team composed of a physician, social worker, ward nurse, occupational or recreational therapist, and psychiatric aide. This program was designed to help residents adjust to the need for hospitalization and to the realities of the aging process. Fitzgerald, Peszke, and Goodwin (1978) and Jacobson (1978) also have discussed the advantages of teamwork in nontraditional mental health settings.

Future Trends

Interdisciplinary teams are fulfilling important functions in both traditional and nontraditional mental health settings. In an era of economic austerity with respect to human services, mental health administrators and planners must scrutinize available mental health resources and devise ways to increase their effectiveness and efficiency. For example, appropriate community supports and services for the severely mentally handicapped must be designed and delivered. Interdisciplinary teams, with the social worker in a key position, can make valuable contributions in this area. As we have seen, mental health teams can also be effectively exploited in a variety of nontraditional areas. To realize the potential of the interdisciplinary approach in the mental health field requires community acceptance, which the social work team member already enjoys, and flexibility on the part of practitioners and training programs.

REFERENCES

BENEDETTO, R. D. "The 23-Hour Bed: Alternative to Hospitalization." *Health and Social Work* 1977, *2*(2):74–88.

BICKFORD, J. H., JR. "Insiders versus Outsiders: Group Ritual in a Mental Health Team." *Hospital and Community Psychiatry* 1974, *25*(11):745–746.

BLOOM, B. L., and PARAD, H. J. "Interdisciplinary Training and Interdisciplinary Functioning: A Survey of Attitudes and Practices in Community Mental Health." *American Journal of Orthopsychiatry* 1976, *46*(4):669–677.

BRILL, N. I. *Teamwork: Working Together in the Human Services.* Philadelphia: Lippincott, 1976.

BURCHILL, E. "Barrow: A Geriatric Treatment Facility." *Advance* 1977, *27*(7): 8–9.

CALLICUTT, J. W. "Milieu Therapy." Lecture presented at the Counseling Center, Bangor, Maine, July 1971.

CHAMBERLIN, H. R. "The Interdisciplinary Team: Contributions by Allied Medical and Nonmedical Disciplines." In S. Gabel and M. T. Erickson (eds.), *Child Development and Developmental Disabilities.* Boston: Little, Brown, 1980.

CHILMAN, C. *Adolescent Sexuality in a Changing American Society.* U.S. Department of Health, Education, and Welfare, Public Health Services 1979.

FITZGERALD, J. F., PESZKE, M. A., and GOODWIN, R. C. "Competency Evaluations in Connecticut." *Hospital and Community Psychiatry* 1978, *29*(7):450–453.

FOLKINS, C., and SPENSLEY, J. "Peer Rating by a Community Mental Health Team: A Positive Approach to Accountability." *American Journal of Orthopsychiatry* 1977, *47*(2):331–335.

GRIEFF, B. S. "The History of Occupational Psychiatry." *Psychiatric Opinion* 1978, *15*(12):10–18.

HALL, J. "Decisions, Decision, Decisions." *Psychology Today* 1971, *5*(6):51.

HIRSCHOWITZ, R. G. "The Able-Stable Model: An Approach to Building Effective Mental Health Teams." *Hospital and Community Psychiatry* 1973, *24*(12):845–846.

JACOBSON, S. B. "A Mental Health Team Approach in a Voluntary Nursing Home." *Gerontological Society* 1978, *18*(5; pt 2):86.

JOHNSON, E., CROCKET, J. T., FREEHLICH, E., and MESSICK, J. M. "Adopting New Models for Continuity of Care: The Ward as Mini-Mental-Health-Center." *Hospital and Community Psychiatry* 1975, *26*(9):601–604.

NEW, P. K. "An Analysis of the Concept of Teamwork." *Community Mental Health Journal* 1968, *4*(4):326–333.

President's Commission on Mental Health. *Report to the President,* vol. 1. Washington, D.C.: U.S. Government Printing Office, 1978.

PUSIĆ, E. "The Administration of Welfare." In F. D. Perlmutter (ed.), *A Design for Social Work Practice.* New York: Columbia University Press, 1974.

SCHWARTZ, S. "Decentralizing a Community Mental Health Center's Service Delivery System." *Hospital and Community Psychiatry* 1974, *25*(11):740-742.

SHAPIRO, E. R., and GUDEMAN, J. E. "Using the Team Concept to Change a Psychoanalytically Oriented Therapeutic Community." *Hospital and Community Psychiatry* 1974, *25*(3):166-169.

SHERR, V. T., and GOFFI, M. T. "On-site Geropsychiatric Services to Guests of Residential Homes." *Journal of the American Geriatrics Society* 1977, *25*(6):269-272.

SMITH, N. F. "Interdisciplinary Training for Community Mental Health Service." *Journal of Education for Social Work* 1974, *10*(2):106-113.

SPENSLEY, J., and LANGSLEY, D. G. "Interdisciplinary Training of Mental Health Professionals." *Journal of Psychiatric Education* 1977, *1*(1):75-84.

STANTON, A. H., and SCHWARTZ, M. S. *The Mental Hospital,* New York: Basic Books, 1954.

U.S. Bureau of the Census. *Special Census Data.* Washington, D.C.: U.S. Government Printing Office, 1975.

CHAPTER 11

Research

Joseph J. Bevilacqua
A. Levond Jones

THE SOCIAL WORK PROFESSION is currently examining its research posture in its professional education efforts and taking stock of its practice patterns in research utilization and production. The record is not encouraging, and more people are becoming aware of its inadequacy. Research findings are poorly utilized in social work practice (Rosenblatt, 1968), and a great distance exists between our scholarship and its application in professional work. We are at best ambivalent about the utility of research, even though, as we will demonstrate, the production of research evidences important subject areas that are pertinent to social work practice.

The mental health setting is also in transition today. Effectiveness of treatment programs, for example, is being questioned, particularly as cost factors in health care are becoming increasingly important. The social dimension of mental health is being rediscovered, with increasing attention devoted to community support, case management and social services. Thus there perhaps has never been a better time for the need for social work to examine its mental health applications.

How social work research has fared in the mental health milieu is the basic question that will guide our discussion. Indeed, is there a body of research that can be identified as social work-related in the mental health field? Are there illustrations of a "best practice model" that can shed light and provide direction for the profession generally? We begin with a brief review of social work research in this area. Next, the social work literature will be examined to determine what patterns, if any, of social work research exist as it relates to mental health. These patterns will be evaluated against current social work practice issues to identify their contribution to the mental health field. Finally, we examine the future of research in light of current government policies.

The Research Dilemma

Historically, research has provided the impetus for social welfare planning and social change, as indicated by the early works of such European social reformers or theorists as John Howard, Frederic LePlay, Charles Booth, and Emile Durkheim (Polansky, 1971). In this country, Dorothea Dix in the 1840s extensively documented the poor treatment of the mentally ill in almshouses and prisons. She brought these data to the attention of various state and federal legislators, with the result that mental hospitals were begun, enlarged, or improved (See Chapter 2).

Though not a social worker, Dix can be credited with the earliest social action research. Such investigations focus on inadequate and deteriorating social conditions; a more sophisticated type of inquiry into social work practice is less well represented in the literature. This lack is important because scientific investigation is one of the hallmarks of a profession. Yet,

social workers . . . don't like to study research; they seldom use research studies in their professional work or to improve their skills; their professional reading is not research oriented; they are not likely to conduct research after leaving school; and they have considerable difficulty accepting research with negative findings. (Rubin and Rosenblatt, 1979, p. 9)

Too often, social workers conceive of research as complex technological quantification with a laboratory overtone. Polansky (1975) has reminded us that social work research concerns itself with all the many areas in which social workers are professionally involved. He defines social work research as follows: "To the extent that an investigator's effort to collect knowledge relevant to social work planning or practice follows the scientific method, it is thought of as social work research" (1971, p. 1099).

In recent years, however, the Council on Social Work Education (CSWE) and the National Association of Social Workers (NASW) with support from the National Institute of Mental Health have sponsored conferences on the ramifications of the paucity of social work research and the corrective actions that need to be taken (Rubin and Rosenblatt, 1979; Fanshel, 1980). Rubin and Rosenblatt (1979) reviewed the causes of this weak research orientation in social work:

1. Intellectual faddism and conflict between segments of the social work profession do not allow for the cumulation of research.
2. Social workers have more of a "people orientation" rather than an interest in abstract knowledge.
3. Tasks and career ladders in the profession do not require practitioners to conduct or use research.

The profession is beginning to address these factors. A nationwide survey of the twenty-two research centers affiliated with graduate schools of social work (SWRCs) found that universities, schools of social work and the social work profession are making unparalleled investments in university-based social work research activities. These investments are reflected in the relatively large number of researchers investigating problems related to social welfare, in the rapid growth in the number of functionally organized SWRCs, and in the volume of public and private financial resources obtained in support of social work research activities. This commitment also is manifested in the willingness of many widely dispersed public and private universities to provide the auspice for an SWRC. The establishment of two new social work research journals also attests to the renewed importance the profession is ascribing to social work's responsibility for generating knowledge. (Estes, 1979, p. 10)

Table 11.1 identifies the current research priorities of the social work research centers.

The gulf between social work research and practice is a prime concern and attention is now focused on bridging that gap. Research should be more relevant to the practice community but it will also have to be used by practitioners. Scott Briar has suggested a speciality of "clinical scientists" (Rubin and Rosenblatt, 1979, p. 21).

Kirk, Osmolov, and Fischer (1976) suggest the following for increasing utilization of research by social workers.

1. Research findings must be relevant to practice.
2. Practical application must be disseminated effectively to potential users.
3. Users need to have skills and incentive to change their professional behavior in accordance with new knowledge.

In summary, the social work profession has traditionally appreciated the value of research to identify social problems. It has failed, however, to integrate research findings into practice and to investigate practices in a rigorous fashion. Training programs have neglected to teach effective research methodologies and consequently the practitioner is both a poor user of research findings and an inadequate investigator. Tentative steps to rectify this situation have been taken, but federal funding cutbacks in the social services threaten the future of social work research.

Social Work Research and Mental Health

Maas's (1978) review of research in the social services discussed major, recent social work investigations in mental health:

Unfortunately, sophistication of design and standardization of method continue to outrun theoretical advance. Most studies can, at best, be described as purely empirical; even those involving "theory of the middle range" never oppose common sense. Social work has imported more in the way of technology than it has of conceptual brilliance from cognate disciplines. This is unfortunate, for—to explicate a saying—the race really goes more often to the swift. We would have

TABLE 11.1
Research Priorities of Social Work Research Centers, 1978*

Focuses of Research	SWRCs Assigning Moderate to High Priority		Studies in Progress		Studies Completed in the Last 24 Months	
	Number	Percentage	Number	Percentage†	Number	Percentage†
Organization of social work						
History	1	6	0	0	1	.5
Manpower	6	33	9	4.9	3	1.5
Social work education and training	14	78	25	13.7	16	8.1
Ethics and values	2	11	1	.5	0	0
Interprofessional relationships	4	22	2	1.1	0	0
Standards and practices	4	22	7	3.8	0	0
Social work organizations and societies	1	6	2	1.1	1	.5
Total			46	25.1	21	10.6
Modes of social work practice						
Services to individuals, families, and groups	6	33	0	0	0	0
Community organization	0	0	1	.5	0	0
Social administration	10	56	10	5.5	13	6.6
Social planning	8	44	2	1.1	0	0

(cont.)

TABLE 11.1 *(Continued)*

Focuses of Research	SWRCs Assigning Moderate to High Priority		Studies in Progress		Studies Completed in the Last 24 Months	
	Number	*Percentage*	*Number*	*Percentage†*	*Number*	*Percentage†*
Social policy analysis	5	28	0	0	1	.5
Research and evaluation	6	33	2	1.1	2	1.0
Consultation	3	17	1	.5	1	.5
Total			16	8.7	17	8.6
Fields of practice						
Aging and aged	14	78	10	5.5	10	5.1
Alcohol and drug addiction	9	50	8	4.4	11	5.6
Crime and delinquency	6	33	13	7.1	28	14.2
Economic security	4	22	1	.5	1	.5
Family and child welfare	15	83	13	7.1	18	9.1
Health and medical care	10	56	10	5.5	6	3.0
Mental health and mental retardation	11	61	11	6.0	13	6.6
Physically handicapped	6	33	9	4.9	11	5.6
Housing and urban development	3	17	0	0	0	0

Early childhood and public education	5	28	7	3.8	23	11.7
Civil rights and civil liberties	0	0	2	1.1	1	.5
Employment and unemployment	6	33	5	2.7	6	3.0
Other (such as International social welfare, white racism, and population control)	3	17	1	.5	6	3.0
Total			90	49.1	134	67.9
Research on special populations						
Poor	9	50	3	1.6	2	1.0
Minorities	10	56	10	5.5	8	4.1
Women	10	56	9	4.9	5	2.5
Youth	8	44	9	4.9	10	5.1
Total			31	16.9	25	12.7
Total all categories			183	100	197	100

Source: Copyright 1979, National Association of Social Workers, Inc. Reprinted with permission, from *Social Work Research & Abstracts*, Vol. 15, No. 2 (Summer 1979), Table 3, pp. 6–7.
*Tabulations based on 18 SWRCs that provided complete data.
†Percentages may not total to 100 because of rounding.

been glad to have encountered more studies involving creative theoretical leaps. But so would every field.

An interesting shift, however, has been in the relatively greater weight placed on studies of how to help and the seeming decline in the volume of studies of etiology, the causes of what is wrong. This is an encouraging and healthy direction, especially when studies go beyond evaluating what has been done to include leads about what might be tried that could be more fruitful. In this connection it seems that the partialization of the helping process into segments lending themselves to thorough investigation is hopeful. (Pp. 189–190)

Social work research in mental health generally appears not in social work journals but in psychiatric periodicals. Occasional studies are reported in interdisciplinary publications like the *American Journal of Orthopsychiatry* and *Hospital and Community Psychiatry*. The more consistent pattern, however, of social work researchers whose full professional efforts are in mental health, is to publish in non-social work publications. A corollary to this is the co-authorship phenomenon where social workers collaborate with other major disciplines, primarily psychiatry and psychology and to a lesser extent nursing.

The profile of social work research in mental health includes: a highly specialized effort, low utilization of social work journals, and collaboration with other disciplines, such as psychiatry, psychology, and nursing. This, of course, suggests a high isolation factor within the social work profession, which clearly has implications for developing the kind of readership that leads to sophisticated utilization and further knowledge development.

Indeed, Polansky and Kent's (in Maas, 1978) review of the literature on individual counseling in the social services purposefully did not limit itself to studies done only by social workers. However, there is utility in attempting to determine if a social work identity does exist in a field which is interdisciplinary in its theoretical perspectives and clinical applications. Mental health represents a very uneven field of practice within the various host disciplines that sustain and nurture its development. This, of course, reflects the larger society where public policies for mental health in the United States are not consistent or clear and at best are treated ambivalently. The social movement of the deinstitutionalization of public mental hospitals during the last twenty years is one example of the ebb and flow of uncertain policy.

However, we suggest that social work research in mental health does constitute an important effort that is distinguished by its emphases on the social environment, social interaction, and social support in its consideration of therapeutic or rehabilitative endeavors.

This approach is well illustrated by Hogarty, Segal, Weissman, Klein, and Linn. They have done interdisciplinary research in the "hard" area of mental illness, i.e., depression, schizophrenia, chronic illness, mental hospital admission and discharge, psychopharmacological studies, community residential placement, and social milieu assessment and analysis. Many of the studies are longitudinal and reflect "hard" science technology in a classic sense, including controlled studies, use of independent raters, attempted double blind conditions, and measurement development through instrumentation.

Hogarty has concentrated on schizophrenia (Hogarty, 1971, 1977, 1979; Hogarty, Goldberg, and Schooler, 1975; Hogarty, Ulrich, Goldberg, and Schooler, 1976). He works in a psychiatric research institute and has been involved with well-controlled investigations of a high technical order. Drugs are an important variable in his research (Hogarty, 1981; Hogarty, Goldberg, and the Collaborative Study Group, 1973; Hogarty, Goldberg, and Schooler, 1974a, 1974b; Hogarty, Schooler, Ulrich, Mussare, Ferro, and Herron, 1979; Hogarty, and Ulrich, 1972, 1977; Hogarty, Ulrich, and Mussare, 1976). These drug studies are creatively informed by Hogarty's professional social work perspective on community supports, admission and discharge (Hogarty, 1966, 1968; Hogarty, Dennis, Guy, and Gross, 1968; Hogarty, and Gross, 1966), foster care, and family therapy. Instrumentation and evaluation protocols have been developed, and both relapsed and nonrelapsed patients have been followed up for several years (Hogarty, 1975, in press; Hogarty, Katz, and Lowery, 1967). Hogarty also has studied day care programs for mental patients, community based care, and hospital care.

Segal's work emphasizes the chronic patient but pays primary attention to the social dimensions of chronicity (Segal and Aviram, 1978). For example, he has studied the community system (Segal, Chandler, and Aviram, 1980), the social features of the environment (Segal and Baumohl, 1980a; Segal, Baumohl, and Moyles, 1980), human service organizations and residential programs (Segal and Everett-Dille, 1980), street life (Segal and Baumohl, 1980b), and social integration (Aviram and Segal, 1973). Segal's research also has addressed policy questions, the role of government in social service provision, and treatment outcomes (Segal, 1972).

Segal's methodology is of the field research type. Epidemiologic assessments, interviews, and analysis of policy documents are integral to his work. While his publications have appeared in social work journals, more often they have been printed in non-social work journals.

Weissman has been one of the most prodigious researchers in mental health. Published widely and frequently, she has concentrated her research interests and efforts on the role of women in a number of areas. This has included sexual roles in depression (Weissman, 1972; Weissman, Fox, and Klerman, 1973; Weissman and Klerman, 1973, 1977a, 1977b; Weissman, Klerman, and Paykel, 1974; Weissman and Myers, 1979, 1980a; Weissman and Paykel, 1972, 1974; Weissman, Paykel, and Klerman, 1972; Weissman, Pincus, and Radding, 1973), and occupations (Weissman, Nelson, and Hackman, 1972). Other work has focused on research methodology (Orvaschel, Sholomskas, and Weissman, 1980; Weissman and Klerman, 1978; Weissman and Meyers, 1980b; Weissman, Orvaschel, and Padian, 1979), as well as issues in social adjustment (Weissman, 1975; Weissman, 1976).

The material cited above is selective. Her work, over time and taken together, is both a significant and interesting commentary on the range of research in mental health and the importance of the psychosocial component in mental illness.

Klein has extensively studied social and environmental variables as predictors of social outcome and community adjustment in chronic schizophrenia. She has been very involved with avoiding and resolving the discharge problems of chronic schizophrenics. Klein has extended her investigations of the chronic schizophrenic's adjustment to the community to include cultural factors: "Family and Community Variables in Adjustment of Turkish and Missouri Schizophrenics" (Klein, Person, Çetingök, and Itil, 1978) has implications for the deinstitutionalization movement. Klein reported that

> certain variables within the family and community . . . make for rehospitalization after discharge. . . . Optimum benefit from psychiatric treatment can be realized only insofar as the social environment can be controlled to meet the [schizophrenic] patient's needs. (P. 246)

Klein has also contributed to research methodology. In her cross-cultural study (Klein et al., 1978), psychiatrists from Missouri and Turkey viewed videotapes to rate symptomatology of schizophrenic patients. The purpose was to determine whether psychiatrists from both cultures would comparably rate patients.

Finally, Klein (Lafferty, Holden, and Klein, 1980), has investigated the relationship between specific norms (proscriptive, prescriptive, and nonscriptive) and chronic alcoholism.

Linn has been concerned with the factors affecting successful aftercare of the deinstitutionalized. In one study, she examined foster home characteristics associated with improved social functioning and found "improved outcome related to more children in the homes, fewer boarders and smaller size" (quoted in Klett and Caffey, 1980, p. 129). She also found a difference in the foster home needs of schizophrenics and nonschizophrenics. Another aftercare study for schizophrenic patients compared the treatment interventions of drug therapy alone or day treatment plus drug therapy (Linn, Caffey, Klett, Hogarty, and Lamb, 1979).

Linn also has developed a social dysfunction rating scale (SDRS), an instrument that can provide a valuable quantitative measure of clients' social dysfunction, and can be of particular use for assessment of treatment change. Evidence of the accuracy of the SDRS as a social measure is provided by Goodman, Schulthorpe, Evje, Slater, and Linn (1969). In this study social worker teams assessed psychiatric and nonpsychiatric outpatients at a VA hospital. One worker used the SDRS, the other employed clinical appraisal for each patient in the sample. It was found that the nature of dysfunction differed between the two patient groups, with the psychiatric group particularly distinguished by emotional withdrawal, adaptive rigidity, lack of participation in the community, goallessness, and low self-concept. The global clinical judgment of one rater correlated highly with the SDRS scores of the patients assessed by the other social worker using the scale.

Linn's research interests also include studies of the geriatric population in the areas of drug abuse, physical illness, and nursing home care. (Lincoln, Berryman, and Linn, 1973; Linn, Linn, and Gurel, 1973; Linn and Gurel, 1969).

Mental Health Manpower Research

A major accomplishment of the National Institute of Mental Health (NIMH) during the late 1970s was to fund a series of grants for studies dealing with mental health manpower development across the nation. This project recognized the important role of the states in mental health manpower activities but did not anticipate the total transfer of support from the federal government to the states that the Reagan administration intends with its block grant policy.

A number of these NIMH-sponsored studies have examined the role of the traditional disciplines in mental health settings. One such project in Rhode Island, representative of a number of manpower studies across the country, was undertaken by the Department of Mental Health, Retardation and Hospitals (MHRH), Division of Human Resource Development (Bevilacqua and Angelini, 1978–1982).

NIMH awarded the department a three-year grant to:

1. develop a comprehensive manpower plan for MHRH
2. participate in key policy decisions in the public and private sectors that related to the acquisition and retention of staff to meet the service needs of clients and patients who were mentally disabled
3. develop a coordinated, comprehensive manpower information system

These projects generally highlighted community patterns of planning, staffing ratios, recruitment and retention policies, professional-political issues, and the organizational dimensions of knowledge development and training, with a high focus on university-practice rating linkages. The project will also study the way the state's institutions of higher education prepare mental health professionals to meet patients' needs and keep current the skills of the practitioner.

The Future of Research

The work of Hogarty, Klein, Linn, Segal, and Weissman, along with broader efforts such as the manpower study described above, are important to the field of social service. How this information is used by social workers is not known. The fact that papers on important studies do not always appear in social work journals is a further important dimension to the profession's poor use of research.

The paucity of "creative theoretical leaps" raised by Polansky and Kent (Maas, 1978) in much of the research they reviewed is confirmed by the "best practice" view we have taken. There clearly is, however, a major contribution to the social dimension of mental illness as seen in the clarification of some of the stereotypical thinking that dominates so much of the field in mental health. The whole question of better understanding of social support and its implications for successful adjustment of the chronic mentally ill patient has emerged from the works of these authors and other social work researchers as well. The clinical condition of treatment, community placement, and the proper use of social support mechanisms all have been enhanced by these efforts.

Social work has begun the enormous task of correcting the imbalances and eliminating the gaps in its research literature. This effort has had some noteworthy success in the mental health field, evident in the work of Hogarty, Klein, and others. Implementation and integration of these research efforts in social work practice has yet to be accomplished.

Meeting these goals is complicated by pressures to reduce public sector services. The Reagan administration's cutbacks of federal support for human services have eliminated virtually all federal funding of social and behavioral research. The role of the federal government, particularly the NIMH, in fostering and supporting social work research in mental health has been critical; its absence will create an incalculable void. Of course, social work practice will also be jeopardized by Reagan's human services policy. Mr. Reagan set this policy when he stated in his 1981 budget message to Congress: "the taxing power of Government . . . must not be used to regulate the economy or bring about social change."

As we have come of age in the recognition of an important role for social work in mental health research, in clinical applications as well as in policy development and assessment, the necessary support for this endeavor is in great jeopardy. Without federal assistance and with reduced private funding likely, the social work profession faces a grave crisis in the years ahead. State and local government cannot provide the necessary support. Undoubtedly, the various disciplines in the human services will have to develop cooperative strategies in order to survive. At the same time, the social work profession will have to take careful stock of its own areas of interest and integrate material and manpower resources in creative and efficient ways. The breadth of review taken by Maas (1966, 1971, 1978) may have to be institutionalized with both the social work educational institutions and the practice fields investing more formally their time, energy, and resources. Without such a common foundation, all of social work research, its many specialties, and the professional practice itself will be essentially flawed.

The lack of a common foundation works against the integration of knowledge into practice, and makes more difficult the necessary connection between the two.

A profession's viability in the end is its ability to legitimize and foster open inquiry relevant to its practice. The lack of this connection dooms the profession to stagnation and, ultimately, the loss of sanction from the larger society.

REFERENCES

AVIRAM, U., and SEGAL, S. P. "Exclusion of the Mentally Ill." *Archives of General Psychiatry* 1973, *29*(1):126-131.

BEVILACQUA, J. J., and ANGELINI, D. E. Unpublished studies, Rhode Island Department of Mental Health, Retardation and Hospitals (NIMH grant 1978–1982), 1-T23-MH-153-93-03-STC.

ESTES, R. J. "Social Work Research Centers." *Social Work Research and Abstracts* 1979, *15*(2):3-16.

FANSHEL, D. (ed.), *Future of Social Work Research.* New York: National Association of Social Workers, 1980.

GOODMAN, S. P., SCHULTHORPE, W. B., EVJE, M., SLATER, P., and LINN, W. "Social Dysfunction among Psychiatric and Non-psychiatric Outpatients." *Journal of the American Geriatrics Society* 1969, *17*(7):694-700.

HOGARTY, G. E. "Discharge Readiness: The Components of a Casework Judgment." *Social Casework* 1966, *47*(3):165-171.

———. "Hospital Differences in the Release of Discharge Ready Chronic Schizophrenics." *Archives of General Psychiatry* 1968, *18*(3):367-372.

———. "The Plight of Schizophrenics in Modern Treatment Programs." *Hospital Community Psychiatry* 1971, *22*(7):197-203.

———. "Informant Ratings of Community Adjustment." In I. Waskow (ed.), *Psychotherapy Change Measures.* Washington, D.C.: U.S. Government Printing Office, 1975.

———. "Treatment and the Course of Schizophrenia." *Schizophrenia Bulletin* 1977, *3*(4):587-599.

———. "Aftercare Treatment of Schizophrenia: Current Status and Future Direction." In H. M. Van Praag (ed.), *Management of Schizophrenia: Biological and Sociological Aspects.* Assen, Netherlands: Van Gorcum, 1979.

———. "Natural and Therapeutic Environmental Indicators of Maintenance Dosage Requirements." *Psychopharmacology Bulletin* 1981, *17*(1):36-37.

HOGARTY, G. E., DENNIS, H., GUY, W., and GROSS, M. "Who Goes There: A Critical Evaluation of Admissions to a Psychiatric Day Hospital." *American Journal of Psychiatry* 1968, *124*(7):934–944.

HOGARTY, G. E., GOLDBERG, S. C., and the Collaborative Study Group. "Drug and Sociotherapy in the Aftercare of Schizophrenic Patients: One-Year Relapse Rates." *Archives of General Psychiatry* 1973, *28*(1):54–64.

HOGARTY, G. E., GOLDBERG, S. C., and SCHOOLER, N. R. "Drug and Sociotherapy in the Aftercare of Schizophrenic Patients. Part II: Two-Year Relapse Rates." *Archives of General Psychiatry* 1974, *31*(5):603–608. (a)

————. "Drug and Sociotherapy in the Aftercare of Schizophrenic Patients. Part III: Adjustment of Non-relapsed Patients." *Archives of General Psychiatry* 1974, *31*(5):609–618. (b)

————. "Drug and Sociotherapy in the Aftercare of Schizophrenia: A Review." In M. Greenblatt (ed.), *Drugs in Combination with Other Therapies*. New York: Grune & Stratton, 1975.

HOGARTY, G. E., and GROSS, M. "Pre-admission Symptom Differences between First Admitted Schizophrenics in the Pre and Post Drug Era." *Comprehensive Psychiatry* 1966, *7*(2):134–140.

HOGARTY, G. E., KATZ, M., and LOWERY, A. "Identifying Candidates from a Normal Population for a Community Mental Health Program." In R. R. Monroe, G. D. Klee, and E. B. Brady (eds.), *Psychiatric Epidemiology and Mental Health Planning*. Washington, D.C.: American Psychiatric Association, 1967.

HOGARTY, G. E., SCHOOLER, N. R., ULRICH, R. F., MUSSARE, F., FERRO, P., and HERRON, E. "Fluphenazine and Social Therapy in the Aftercare of Schizophrenic Patients: Relapse Analyses of a Two-Year Controlled Trial." *Archives of General Psychiatry* 1979, *36*(12):1283–1294.

HOGARTY, G. E., and ULRICH, R. F. "The Discharge Readiness Inventory." *Archives of General Psychiatry* 1972, *26*(5):419–426.

————. "Temporal Effects of Drug and Placebo in Delaying the Relapse of Schizophrenic Patients." *Archives of General Psychiatry* 1977, *34*(3):297–301.

HOGARTY, G. E., ULRICH, R. F., GOLDBERG, S., and SCHOOLER, N. "Sociotherapy and the Prevention of Relapse among Schizophrenic Patients: An Artifact of Drug?" In R. Spitzer and D. Klein (eds.), *Evaluation of Psychological Therapies*. Baltimore: Johns Hopkins Press, 1976.

HOGARTY, G. E., ULRICH, R. F., and MUSSARE, F. "Drug Discontinuation among Long Term Successfully Treated Schizophrenic Outpatients." *Diseases of the Nervous System,* 1976, *37*(9):494–500.

KIRK, A., OSMOLOV, J., and FISCHER, J. "Social Workers' Involvement in Research." *Social Work* 1976, *21*(2):121–124.

KLEIN, H. E., PERSON, T. M., ÇETINGÖK, M., and ITIL, T. M. "Family and Community Variables in Adjustment of Turkish and Missouri Schizophrenics." *Comprehensive Psychiatry* 1978, *19*(3):233–240.

KLETT, C., and CAFFEY, M., JR. "Foster Home Characteristics and Psychiatric Patient Outcome." *Archives of General Psychiatry* 1980, *37*(2):129.

LAFFERTY, N. A., HOLDEN, J. M., and KLEIN, H. E. "Norm Qualities and Alcoholism." *International Journal of Social Psychiatry* 1980, *26*(3):159–166.

LINCOLN, L., BERRYMAN, M., and LINN, M. W. "Drug Abuse: A Comparison of Attitudes." *Journal of Comparative Psychiatry* 1973, *14*(5):465–471.

LINN, B. S., LINN, M. W., and GUREL, L. "Correlates of Prognosis: A Study of the Physician's Clinical Judgement." *Medical Care,* 1973 *11*(5):430–434.

LINN, M. W., CAFFEY, E. M., KLETT, J. C., HOGARTY, G., and LAMB, H. R. "Day Treatment and Psychotropic Drugs in Aftercare of Schizophrenic Patients." *Archives of General Psychiatry* 1979, *36*(10):1055–1066.

LINN, M. W., and GUREL, L. "Initial Reactions to Nursing Home Placement." *Journal of the American Geriatric Society* 1969, *17*(2):219–220.

MAAS, H. S. (ed.). *Five Fields of Social Service.* New York: National Association of Social Workers, 1966.

———. (ed.). *Research in the Social Services: A Five-Year Review.* New York: National Association of Social Workers, 1971.

———. (ed.). *Social Service Research: Review of Studies* New York: National Association of Social Workers, 1978.

"The Mental Health Disciplines." *Journal of Hospital and Community Psychiatry* 1976, *27*(7):498.

ORVASCHEL, H., SHOLOMSKAS, D., and WEISSMAN, M. M. "The Assessment of Psychopathology and Behavioral Problems in Children: A Review of Scales Suitable for Epidemiological and Clinical Research (1967–1969)." In *Mental Health System Reports.* CHHS pub. no. (ADM) 80-1037. Rockville, Md.: Alcohol, Drug Abuse, and Mental Health Administration, 1980.

POLANSKY, N. "Research in Social Work." In R. Morris (ed.), *Encyclopedia of Social Work* (16th ed.), vol. 2. New York: National Association of Social Workers, 1971.

POLANSKY, N. (ed.). *Social Work Research.* Chicago: University of Chicago Press, 1975.

ROSENBLATT, A. "The Practitioner's Use and Evaluation of Research." *Social Work,* 1968, *13*(1):53–59.

RUBIN, A., and ROSENBLATT, A. (eds.). *Sourcebook on Research Utilization.* New York: Council on Social Work Education, 1979.

SEGAL, S. P. "Research on the Outcome of Social Work Therapeutic Interventions: A Review of the Literature." *Journal of Health and Social Behavior* 1972, *13*(1):3–17.

SEGAL, S. P., and AVIRAM, U. *The Mentally Ill in Community-Based Sheltered Care: A Study of Community Care and Social Integration.* New York: Wiley, 1978.

SEGAL, S. P., and BAUMOHL, J. "Engaging the Disengaged: Proposals on Madness and Vagrancy." *Social Work* 1980, *25*(5):358–365. (a)

———. "Factors in the Receipt of Therapeutic Assistance in Community Care." *Social Science and Medicine,* 1980, *14A*(6):581–587. (b)

SEGAL, S. P., BAUMOHL, J., and MOYLES, E. M. "Neighborhood Types and Community Reaction to the Mentally Ill: A Paradox of Intensity." *Journal of Health and Social Behavior* 1980, *21*(4):345–359.

SEGAL, S. P., CHANDLER, S., and AVIRAM, U. "Antipsychotic Drugs in Community-Based Sheltered-Care Homes." *Social Science and Medicine* 1980, *14A*(6): 589–596.

SEGAL, S. P., and EVERETT-DILLE, L. *Coping Styles and Factors in Male/Female Social Integration.* Berkeley: School of Social Welfare, University of California, 1980.

WEISSMAN, M. M. "The Depressed Woman: Recent Psychosocial Research." *Social Work* 1972, *17*(5):19–26.

———. "The Assessment of Social Adjustment: A Review of Techniques." *Archives of General Psychiatry* 1975, *32*(3):357–365.

———. "Self-destructive Youth: A Problem in Primary Prevention." *Current Concepts in Psychiatry* 1976, *2*(1):2–4.

———. "The Psychological Treatment of Depression: Research Evidence for the Efficacy of Psychotherapy Alone, in Comparison with, and in Combination with Pharmacotherapy." *Archives of General Psychiatry* 1979, *36*(11):1261–1269.

WEISSMAN, M. M., FOX, K., and KLERMAN, G. L. "Hostility and Depression Associated with Suicide Attempts." *American Journal of Psychiatry* 1973, *130*(4):450–455.

WEISSMAN, M. M., and KLERMAN, G. L. "Psychotherapy with Depressed Women: Empirical Study of Content Themes and Reflection." *British Journal of Psychiatry* 1973, *123*:55–61.

———. "The Chronic Depressive in the Community: Unrecognized and Poorly Treated." *Comprehensive Psychiatry* 1977, *18*(6):523–532. (a)

———. "Sex Differences and the Epidemiology of Depression." *Archives of General Psychiatry* 1977, *34*(1):98–111.

———. "Epidemiology of Mental Disorders: Emerging Trends." *Archives of General Psychiatry* 1978, *35*(6):705–712.

WEISSMAN, M. M., KLERMAN, G. L., PAYKEL, E. S., PRUSOFF, B., and HANSON, B. "Treatment Effects on the Social Adjustment of Depressed Patients." *Archives of General Psychiatry* 1974, *30*(6):771–778.

WEISSMAN, M. M., and MYERS, J. K. "Depression in the Elderly: Research Directions in Psychopathology, Epidemiology, and Treatment." *Journal of Geriatric Psychiatry* 1979, *12*(2):187–201.

———. "The Magnitude of Depression in the Community: Who Is Being Treated, by Whom, How, and to What Extent?" *Rhode Island Medical Journal* 1980, *63*(4):109–112. (b)

———. "Psychiatric Disorders in a U.S. Community: The Application of Research Diagnostic Criteria to a Resurveyed Community Sample." *Acta Psychiatrica Scandinovica* 1980, *62*(2):99–111. (c)

WEISSMAN, M. M., NELSON, K., HACKMAN, J., PINCUS, C., and FRUSOC, B. "The Faculty Wife: Her Academic Interests and Qualifications." *American Association of University Professors Bulletin* 1972, 58(3):278–291.

WEISSMAN, M. M., ORVASCHEL, H., and PADIAN, N. *Comparison of Results from Psychiatric Diagnostic, Symptom, and Social Functioning Scales Administered to Children: Technical Report of a Pilot Study.* Rockville, Md.: Alcohol, Drug Abuse, and Mental Health Administration, 1979.

WEISSMAN, M. M., and PAYKEL, E. S. *The Depressed Woman: A Study of Social Relationships.* Chicago: University of Chicago Press, 1974.

———. "Moving and Depression in Women." *Society* 1972, *9*(9):24–28.

WEISSMAN, M. M., PAYKEL, E. S., and KLERMAN, G. L. "The Depressed Woman as a Mother." *Social Psychiatry* 1972, *7*(1):98–108.

WEISSMAN, M. M., PINCUS, C., RADDING, N., LAWRENCE, R., and SIEGEL, R. "The Educated Housewife: Mild Depression and the Search for Work." *American Journal of Orthopsychiatry* 1973, *43*(4):565–573.

Epilogue

James W. Callicutt
Pedro J. Lecca

THE 1980s do not represent the golden era of the human services. To the contrary, in this time of fiscal restraint, cutbacks in social programs and realignment of governmental responsibilities in the mental health arena are rampant. Yet, the incidence of mental health problems is unlikely to decrease. What, then, does this climate signal for the provision of mental health services? Furthermore, what does it portend for the role of social workers in mental health services? Responses to the questions are at best tentative.

First, in the realm of social policy we are witnessing a retreat from the premise that caused the National Institute of Mental Health to be established in 1948 as part of the U.S. Public Health Service. The federal government appears to be renouncing the concept that mental illness and disability are public health concerns that require nationally generated initiatives, incentives, and mental health policy goals. If this trend continues, what state and local provisions will be made for mental health services?

One possible scenario would see increased utilization of state hospitals and other long-term custodial institutions and a concomitant shrinking of services provided by community mental health centers. This would be a complete reversal of the trend outlined in Chapter 2. Indeed, we might see no coherent national mental health policy but, instead, fifty state variations as a result of *presumed* fiscal conservatism regarding the provision of human services. We challenge this presumption: institutional care, compared to community based care, is both financially more expensive and socially more disruptive, hampering patient-community adjustment and functioning.

However, we anticipate another scenario. This one will find community mental health services retrenching temporarily. State hospitals will not reassume a preeminent role in the mental health system. We suspect that the pendulum will swing back and that the federal government will again take

239

an active part in formulating and promoting a national mental health policy. This turnabout will rest, in part, on the recognition that patients can be treated more effectively in the community at costs that are significantly lower than the costs of institutional care. Rising pressures on the institutions, in terms of increased expectations for patient care and treatment, along with renewed awareness of the pervasiveness and magnitude of mental health problems, will stimulate federal government initiatives in this area.

Continued concern with costs is certain. However, in our view, there must be a rethinking of service and funding priorities. As Mechanic (1980) observed:

> Priorities always depend on values; two paramount values are ordinarily applied in thinking about mental health needs. The first is a humanitarian value—the concept of *need;* it is based on the idea that the best services should be made available to those who need them despite the cost, the difficulty in obtaining them, or the pressure on resources. The second concept—the notion of *gain*— is based on the idea that services should be made available when the result achieved is equal to the investment. (Pp. 34–35)

Policy decisions on funding will be incremental in nature rather than radical (see Chapter 2). Our fiscal resources are indeed finite and competition over scarce resources in the human services (as well as defense, international aid, etc.) will require the establishment of priorities. It appears that services to the mentally disabled (chronic) patient will be continued and perhaps strengthened. Professionals, legislators, and volunteers agree about meeting this need, but how this need will be met is another matter. Community mental health centers and total care institutions such as state hospitals will compete over funds until the long-range cost-effectiveness of community based services, compared to institutional services, is recognized.

A number of trends will lead us into the next decade:

- proliferation of prevention programs, health maintenance organizations, and wellness centers
- increased reliance on ambulatory care centers and outpatient clinics
- intensified competition among counselors and psychotherapists in private practice for the mental health client
- short-term resurgence of institutional care at the expense of community based services
- increased attention to community education
- greater reliance on brief therapies, crisis intervention, and stress management
- expanded use of self-help groups

We expect also that social workers in the mental health field will:

- continue to fill administrative, clinical, and research positions in institutional and community based services
- assume leadership roles in designing, developing, administering, and evaluating new mental health services that are not located in hospitals
- be involved more directly in interdisciplinary research projects, especially those that address family dynamics
- continue to struggle against the socioeconomic and cultural barriers that exclude the poor and racial minorities from access to the mental health system
- participate in the development of service integration schemes to facilitate community adjustment of deinstitutionalized individuals
- provide consultation services and encourage the development of social support systems
- employ a wider range of intervention and counseling techniques more effectively to address specific problems

Human problems, including those in the area of mental health, cannot be expected to decline in either severity or number in the foreseeable future. The potential consequences of these problems are staggering to contemplate. Thus, the need for mental health workers will not diminish in the long run despite the short-term economic effects of reduced funding. In fact, we think that there will be an increased need for mental health personnel, especially those having a psychosocial knowledge base that includes understanding of the social environment and community dynamics. At the same time, cuts in the Health Professions Education Assistance Act will have a negative impact on mental health professional training programs throughout the country, possibly resulting in increased use of practitioners such as social workers to fill the gap. Finally, we contend that practice in the mental health arena will continue to provide exciting career opportunities for professionals, including social workers, especially those who are trained in a multimethods approach that embraces administration, planning, community organization, direct practice, and research.

REFERENCES

KAHN, A. J. *Social Policy and Social Services.* New York: Random House, 1973.
MECHANIC, D. *Mental Health and Social Policy.* Englewood Cliffs: Prentice-Hall, 1980.

Glossary

Administration: generic process that includes the planning, development (both organizational and programmatic), budgeting, and evaluation of all organizational activities.

Aftercare: continuing treatment and rehabilitation provided in the community to help the patient adjust following a period of hospitalization.

Behavior therapy: treatment designed to modify the patient's behavior directly rather than inquire into dynamic causes. Typically, the psychopathology is conceptualized as maladaptive behavior. The treatment techniques are adapted from laboratory investigations of learning and may use principles of classical, instrumental, and traumatic avoidance conditioning; reciprocal inhibition and desensitization; simple extinction, etc.

Board of directors: a policymaking body for a non-governmental health or social welfare agency or organization.

Catchment area: geographic area for which a mental health facility has responsibility.

Certificate of need: the National Health Planning and Resources Development Act of 1975 requires state health planning agencies to administer a certificate of need program. The program is concerned with the allocation of capital expenditures, the offering of new institutional health services, and the addition of major medical equipment. After determining the need for proposed allocations, services, and additions, the state health planning agency may issue a certificate of need or deny the request.

Citizen participation: process through which the whole community or a specific constituency participates in the policymaking and governance tasks of an organization.

Clinical administrator: mental health professional, trained primarily in clinical skills, who assumes an administrative function within a human service organization.

Cognitive dissonance: a theory of psychological processes (within the individual) based on the notions "that the simultaneous existence of cognitions which in one way or another do not fit together (dissonance) leads to effort on the part of the person to somehow make them fit better (dissonance reductions)." (quoted from Festinger, L., and Aronson, E. "The Arousal and Reduction of Dissonance in Social Contexts." In D. Cartwright and A. Zander (eds.), *Groups Dynamics*. Evanston: Row, Peterson, 1960 .

Community mental health center: community or neighborhood based facility, or network of facilities, for the prevention and treatment of mental illness, ideally with emphasis on a comprehensive range of services and with convenient access to the population it serves. Since 1964, regulations governing federal support for community centers have required that centers offer at least five services: inpatient, outpatient, partial hospitalization, and emergency services; and consultation and education. Many centers also provide diagnostic, rehabilitative, precare, and aftercare services; offer training; and conduct research.

Community support services: system of services designed for the seriously or chronically mentally disabled to prevent their admission to mental health institutions or to facilitate their discharge into, and adjustment within, a stable and supportive environment.

Contingency planning: process of determining the priority system that will be used in designating the functions, services, and personnel to be eliminated and those be preserved in the face of budget reductions.

Continuity of care: provision of a range of services, geared to client problems of varying degrees of severity, so that clients can move from one service to another with minimal disruption as their needs change in the course of treatment.

Culture of poverty: cluster of factors that combine to create the second-class status of minorities. These factors are low income, unemployment, underemployment, undereducation, poor housing, prejudice, discrimination, cultural and linguistic barriers, and powerlessness.

Day care: part-time service offered by many state mental hospitals, psychiatric departments of general hospitals, private psychiatric facilites, and community mental health and mental retardation centers. Usually the service includes a structured therapeutic program, under supervision, during the day or early evening.

Empathy: feeling *with* another person; that is, entering into the emotional experience of another.

Executive director: chief executive of a health or social welfare agency or organization. May or may not be a clinical administrator.

Gestalt psychology: psychological orientation that stresses the whole person.

Gestalt therapy: psychotherapy that focuses on the integration of the various aspects of the client's experience, including physical sensations, thoughts, feelings, and behavior.

Halfway house: residence for mental patients who do not require hospitalization but do need support and services before returning to fully independent community living.

Health systems agency (HSA): regional agency that is responsible for comprehensive health planning in a specific geographic area. Each HSA within a state works closely with the staff of the state health planning agency.

Hispanic: of Chicano, Puerto Rican, Cuban or other Latin American descent.

Homeostasis: tendency of a social system to remain in a stable state of dynamic equilibrium. Family systems have a powerful tendency to remain at a stable level of functioning and to resist change, which helps maintain a sense of continuity and identity among members.

Insight: awareness of one's motives and reactions.

Intrapsychic: originating from, or taking place within, the psyche.

Introspective: turning one's attention inward to examine one's own feelings.

Length of stay: number of days an individual remains on a particular service—usually an inpatient service. The average length of stay for a hospital usually is the length of stay (in days) for all patients, divided by the total number of patients hospitalized during a given period.

Management: specification of organizational objectives and deployment or organizational resources, both human and fiscal, to achieve organizational goals.

Management information system: manual or automated system for collecting and organizing data on finances, staff activity, client characteristics, and clinical services in a manner that allows for efficient analysis and effective decisionmaking.

Medical model: approach to treatment that views mental health problems as diseases with medical causes and therefore amenable to medical interventions.

Mental health: state of being, relative rather than absolute, in which a person has effected a reasonably satisfactory integration of his/her instinctual drives. This integration is acceptable to the person and his/her social milieu, as reflected in his/her interpersonal relationships, level of satisfaction in living, actual achievements, flexibility, etc.

Middle management: group of senior clinical administrators with responsibility for managing service programs; this group reports to the executive director of the organization.

Morphogenesis: ability of a social system to alter its existing dynamic state of equilibrium. Family systems have the ability to change their ways of operating when new life circumstances occur (birth of a child, change of job, etc.).

Morphostasis: self-correcting process used by a social system to maintain its stable, dynamic equilibrium. As the system encounters new inputs and begins to change, morphostatic mechanisms react to move the system back to its original steady state. Family systems tend to resist change and to maintain long-standing ways of functioning.

Operational: process of defining organizational goals and determining the resources required to achieve them.

Organic brain syndrome: disorder caused by, or associated with, impairment of brain tissue function. Manifestations include disorientation, loss of memory, and difficulty learning or making judgments. The syndrome may be psychotic or nonpsychotic; mild, moderate, or severe.

Paradoxical intervention: therapeutic strategy in which dysfunctional behavior is prescribed; for instance, a family may be directed by the therapist to exaggerate maladaptive patterns. The rationale is that the resistant family will resist the directive and be forced to change; the compliant family, by fulfilling the directive, will demonstrate their control over both the system's functioning and the problem behavior.

Personnel management: recruitment of qualified staff, supervision and evaluation of workers, administration of personnel policies and procedures, and implementation of wage and salary guidelines—all in accordance with federal laws on equal opportunity.

Planning: process of collecting and analyzing information in order to assist the determination of organizational goals and priorities.

Program budgeting: accounting process that allocates funds to specific services and helps to assess a program's fiscal effectiveness.

Social system: conceptual method of describing the means by which a social unit (individual, group, organization, or agency) functions both internally and in relation to other systems.

Social work: use of community resources and of the conscious adaptive capacities of individuals and groups to better the adjustment of an individual to his/her environment and to improve the quality of that environment.

Sociopsychological: social *and* psychological.

Systems theory: conceptualization emphasizing transactions among persons (or organizations) with a defined environment, and the persons (or organizations) in that environment with other surrounding enivronments.

Index